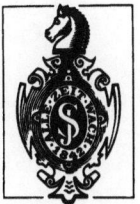

Idiopathic Hydronephrosis

Edited by

P.H. O'Reilly and J.A. Gosling

Foreword by E. Charlton Edwards

With 87 Figures

Springer-Verlag
Berlin Heidelberg New York 1982

P.H. O'Reilly, MD, FRCS,
Consultant Urological Surgeon,
Stepping Hill Hospital,
Stockport, SK2 7JE, England

J.A. Gosling, MD,
Professor of Anatomy,
The Medical School,
University of Manchester,
Oxford Road,
Manchester M13 9PT, England

ISBN-13:978-1-4471-3110-6   e-ISBN-13:978-1-4471-3108-3
DOI: 10.1007/978-1-4471-3108-3

Typeset by Photo-graphics, Stockland, Honiton, Devon

2128/3916-543210

Foreword

For more than a century, the condition now known as *Idiopathic Hydronephrosis* has been recognised as a clinical entity, and following the original description by Rayer in 1841 a variety of procedures were devised in attempts to correct the condition surgically. Most of these early methods were introduced in the last decade of the nineteenth century by several illustrious clinicians, including Trendelenburg, Küster, Fenger and Sutton. For many years diagnosis was based purely upon the patients presenting signs and symptoms and not until the early part of this century was technology available to assist in the pre-operative diagnosis of the condition. Early methods depended upon radiological techniques, and the introduction of the retrograde pyelogram by Voelcker and Lichtenberg in 1906 represented a significant advance in diagnostic methodology. Other methods also dependent upon radiographic techniques were subsequently introduced, including urography in the late 1930s by Swick, and more recently, the method of cineradiography, as pioneered with considerable success by Peter Narath in the decade following World War II.

During the past 50 years a variety of surgical procedures have been introduced for the treatment of idiopathic hydronephrosis. That so many different methods have been devised suggests that no one specific technique is capable of achieving a complete cure in all cases. In practice, most urologists adopt one particular method with which they feel satisfied given that the postoperative results of that particular method are not inferior to those of an alternative procedure. The methods which have been devised and which remain as alternatives in the surgical management of the disease include the intubated ureterostomy originally devised by Davis in 1943. A method attempting to denervate the pelvis and ureter was described by Oldham, but this procedure is rarely practised by present-day urologists. Similarly the nephropexy procedure developed by Hamilton Stewart has fallen from favour, leaving the Foley-Schwyzer Y-V plasty, the spiral flap method of Culp, and the Anderson-Hynes dismembered pyeloureterostomy as the most popular techniques in the surgical treatment of idiopathic hydronephrosis.

Until the early 1960s the causal mechanisms which underlie idiopathic hydronephrosis were largely unknown. However, during the past 10 years considerable advances in our understanding of the condition have taken place. This progress has been achieved largely through a multidisciplinary approach to the study of the normal and abnormal upper urinary tract. This increase in knowledge has in no small part been dependent upon the introduction of modern techniques which have refined the information which can now be obtained from patients with the disease. In recognition of these considerable advances during the past decade, workers in several different fields, but all sharing a common interest in idiopathic hydronephrosis, attended a symposium devoted to the condition. The gathering was organised under the auspices of the Manchester and North West Region Kidney Research Association and held in September 1980 in Manchester, England.

This volume grew out of, and represents extension of, that symposium and contains an up-to-date account of the current state of knowledge on various aspects of idiopathic hydronephrosis. The authors have expanded their contributions to that meeting and their articles have been compiled by the Editors into this single volume (which, incidentally, is the first for over 15 years to be published dealing specifically with this topic). Anyone with an interest in hydronephrosis, whether basic scientist or practising clinician, will find something of interest in the publication. It is certain that the contents of this collection of articles will act as a factual base from which future research will develop and thereby assist further progress in the diagnosis and treatment of this condition.

Manchester, October 1981   E. Charlton Edwards
                                                   MD, MCh, FRCS, FRCSE

Contents

10. Clinical Management

Contributors

C.E. Constantinou Ph.D.
Assistant Professor of Surgery, Division of Urology, Stanford University Medical Center, Stanford, California, USA.

J.S. Dixon B.Sc., Ph.D.
Senior Lecturer in Histology, Department of Anatomy, University of Manchester Medical School, Oxford Road, Manchester M13 9PT, England.

J.C. Djurhuus M.D., Ph.D.
Associate Professor of Experimental Surgery, Department of Urology, Aarhus Kommunehospital, Aarhus, Denmark.

J.A. Gosling M.B., Ch.B., M.D.
Professor of Anatomy, University of Manchester Medical School, Oxford Road, Manchester M13 9PT, England.

J.H. Johnston F.R.C.S., F.R.C.S.I., F.A.C.S.
Consultant Urological Surgeon, Alder Hey Children's Hospital, Liverpool, England.

S.A. Koff M.D.
Assistant Professor of Surgery, Chief, Paediatric Urology Service, University of Michigan Medical Center, Ann Arbor, Michigan, USA.

E.W. Lupton M.D., F.R.C.S.
Senior Registrar in Urology, Manchester Royal Infirmary, Manchester M13 9WL, England.

P.H. O'Reilly M.D., F.R.C.S.
Consultant Urological Surgeon, Stepping Hill Hospital, Stockport SK2 7JE, England.

R.C. Pfister M.D.
Associate Professor of Radiology, Harvard Medical School. Head, Genitourinary Section, Department of Radiology, Massachusetts General Hospital, Boston, Massachusetts, USA.

T. Sherwood F.F.R., F.R.C.R., M.R.C.P., D.C.H.

Professor of Radiology, University of Cambridge and Addenbrookes Hospital, Cambridge, England.

R.H. Whitaker M.Ch., F.R.C.S.

Consultant Urologist, Addenbrookes Hospital, Cambridge, England.

1. The Structure of the Normal and Hydronephrotic Upper Urinary Tract

J.A. Gosling and J.S. Dixon

The aim of this chapter is to provide a brief review of the structure of the upper urinary tract, based on light and electron microscope observations of normal human postoperative material. This description is followed by an account of the morphological changes which occur in the proximal dilated portion of the urinary tract in cases of idiopathic hydronephrosis. It is hoped that these anatomical studies will complement the physiological and clinical investigations described in subsequent chapters, and provide for a better understanding of the functional anomalies which occur in this relatively common condition.

Structure of the Normal Upper Urinary Tract

Histologically the wall of the upper urinary tract comprises three layers; namely, an inner mucosal layer (consisting of urothelium and its supporting lamina propria), a muscular layer, and an outer adventitial layer of connective tissue. The most important component relating to urine transport is the muscle coat and it is to this that particular attention is directed. Significant differences occur in the architecture of the musculature within the wall of the calyces, pelvis, and ureter. Two morphologically and histochemically distinct types of smooth muscle cell are present in certain regions of the upper urinary tract. One type appears similar to smooth muscle found elsewhere, while the other possesses a number of unusual features and herein is referred to as 'atypical' smooth muscle. The distribution of these two types of smooth muscle will now be described.

Distribution of Atypical Smooth Muscle Cells

Atypical smooth muscle cells occur in the region of attachment of each minor calyx to the renal parenchyma. These morphologically distinctive cells are not arranged into compact bundles but instead form a thin sheet of muscle which covers each minor calyceal fornix (Fig. 1.1). These smooth muscle cells also extend across the renal parenchyma which lies between the renal attachments of the minor calyces. Thus, each minor calyx is in effect connected to its neighbours by a thin layer of atypical smooth muscle. In the wall of each minor calyx, atypical smooth muscle cells are arranged longitudinally and form a discrete layer confined to the inner aspect of the muscle coat. This inner layer is closely applied to and interconnects with the bundles of typical smooth muscle (see below). This arrangement continues throughout the walls of the major calyces and renal pelvis (Fig. 1.2). However, in the pelviureteric region this configuration ceases so that the proximal ureter is devoid of a morphologically distinct inner layer (Fig. 1.3). Individually, atypical

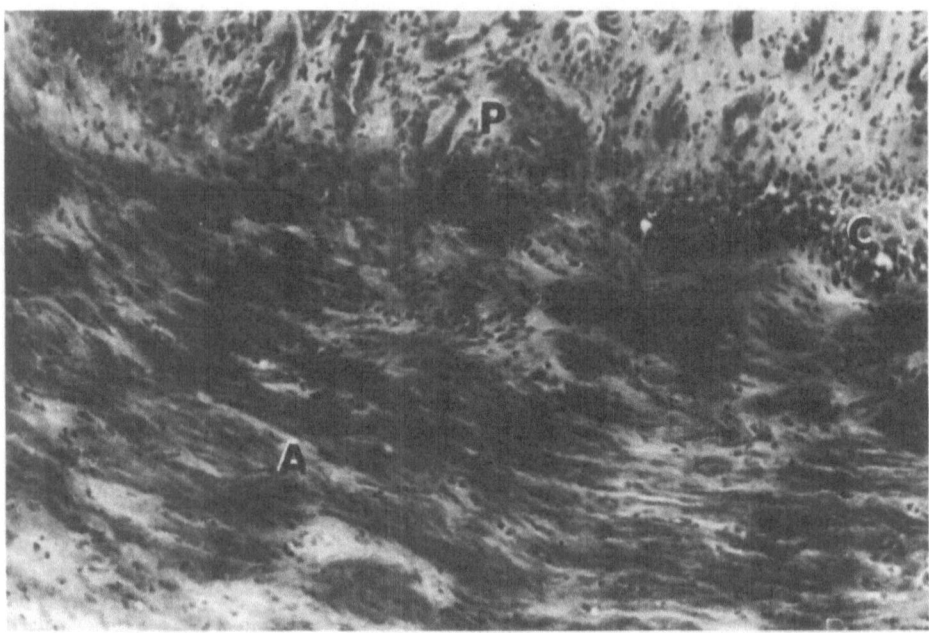

Fig. 1.1. Atypical smooth muscle cells (*A*) form a meshwork which overlies the renal parenchyma (*P*) and extends into the wall of the minor calyx (*C*). (×250)

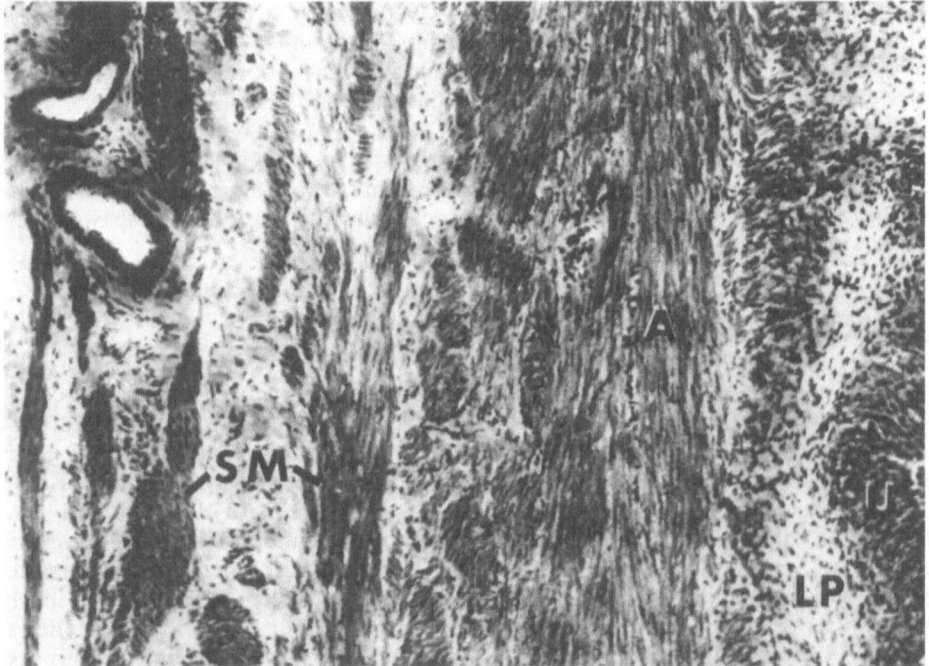

Fig. 1.2. Section through the wall of the renal pelvis. Compact bundles of smooth muscle (*SM*) occur on the outer aspect of the muscle coat. Numerous atypical cells form a layer on the inner aspect (*A*). *U*, urothelium; *LP*, lamina propria. (×150)

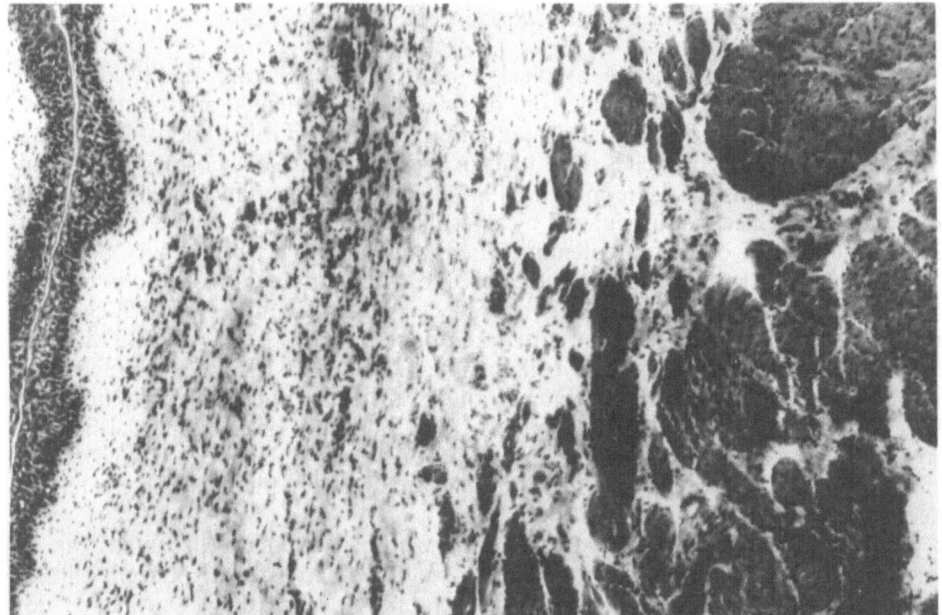

Fig. 1.3. The muscle coat of the ureter consists of irregularly-arranged bundles of smooth muscle cells, widely separated by connective tissue. Note the absence of an inner layer of morphologically distinct (atypical) smooth muscle cells.($\times 100$)

cells are separated from one another for much of their length by quantities of connective tissue. In addition, histochemical studies have shown that these cells differ from typical upper urinary tract smooth muscle in that they are devoid of non-specific cholinesterase. Although the physiological significance of this intracellular enzyme is not known at present, it is a useful means by which to distinguish the two types of smooth muscle cell.

Distribution of Typical Smooth Muscle Cells

Typical spindle-shaped smooth muscle cells are grouped together into compact bundles which are first in evidence in the distal part of each minor calyx. These bundles lie external to the atypical muscle cell layer and extend throughout the major calyces and renal pelvis. In the pelviureteric region these bundles are directly continuous with those which form the muscle coat of the ureter (Fig. 1.3). In the major calyces and renal pelvis these muscle bundles are closely related on their inner aspects to the layer of atypical smooth muscle. Individual bundles lie in various directions although the majority tend to be circularly disposed. These compact bundles of smooth muscle frequently branch and connect with adjacent muscle fascicles, thus forming a plexiform arrangement of inter-communicating muscle bundles. In the pelviureteric region there is no localised thickening of muscle, so that a pelviureteric sphincter cannot be anatomically recognised. The smooth muscle cells forming the muscle bundles of the ureter and also the outer layer of the muscle coat of the renal pelvis and major calyces are rich in non-specific cholinesterase and are easily distinguished from the atypical cell layer.

Fine Structure of Atypical Smooth Muscle Cells

In the electron microscope the atypical smooth muscle cells are readily identified because of their wide separation from one another by collagen and elastic fibrils. Individual cells are extremely elongated and irregular in outline and often possess lateral protrusions or branches (Fig. 1.4). In addition many cells possess rounded or angular projections of sarcoplasm (Fig. 1.5), which enhance their irregular appearance. Each cell is surrounded by a basal lamina, which is often discontinuous over those regions of the sarcolemma where angular projections occur. Caveolae (flask-shaped micropinocytotic vesicles) do not occur in such projections but are present at other regions of the cells' surfaces. The myofilaments of such cells are identical in type to those found in other upper urinary tract smooth muscle. However, within each cell the myofilaments are frequently arranged in elongated bundles separated by areas containing granular reticulum and small mitochondria. This contrasts with their arrangement in typical smooth muscle cells, in which the myofilaments generally occupy the major part of the sarcoplasm (see below). Many of the atypical cells possess areas within their sarcoplasm which contain clusters of electron-dense glycogen granules.

Frequently an elongated sarcoplasmic projection from one cell extends out to form an intercellular junction with a similar protuberance from an adjacent cell. At the junctional region the opposing cell membranes are separated by a gap of not more than 20 nm without any intervening basal lamina (Fig. 1.6). Junctions of this type are similar to the regions of close approach that occur between ureteric smooth muscle cells.

Fine Structure of Typical Smooth Muscle Cells

As described above the outer aspect of the muscle coat of the calyceal and pelvic wall consists of smooth muscle arranged into compact bundles. Such bundles are composed of closely apposed smooth muscle cells separated from their neighbours by relatively little intervening connective tissue (Fig. 1.7). Each smooth muscle cell possesses sarcoplasm packed with longitudinally orientated myofilaments together with numerous electron-dense bodies. Mitochondria are scattered at random throughout the sarcoplasm while scant granular reticulum and Golgi membranes tend to cluster at either pole of the single, elongated nucleus. Rows of caveolae interspersed with electron-dense regions are observed at the sarcolemma of each smooth muscle cell. Individual smooth muscle cells are surrounded by a basal lamina except at regions of close approach where a gap of 15–20 nm separates adjacent cell membranes in the absence of intervening basal lamina material. Such regions are frequently observed between adjacent smooth muscle cells within a muscle bundle. Apart from such regions, the narrow intercellular spaces contain occasional collagen fibres while elastic fibres are very rarely observed.

Innervation of the Upper Urinary Tract

Autonomic nerve fibres occur in the muscle coat of the calyceal wall, the renal pelvis and the ureter. However, the majority of such nerves accompany small blood vessels which run through the muscle layer to supply a rich capillary plexus in the lamina

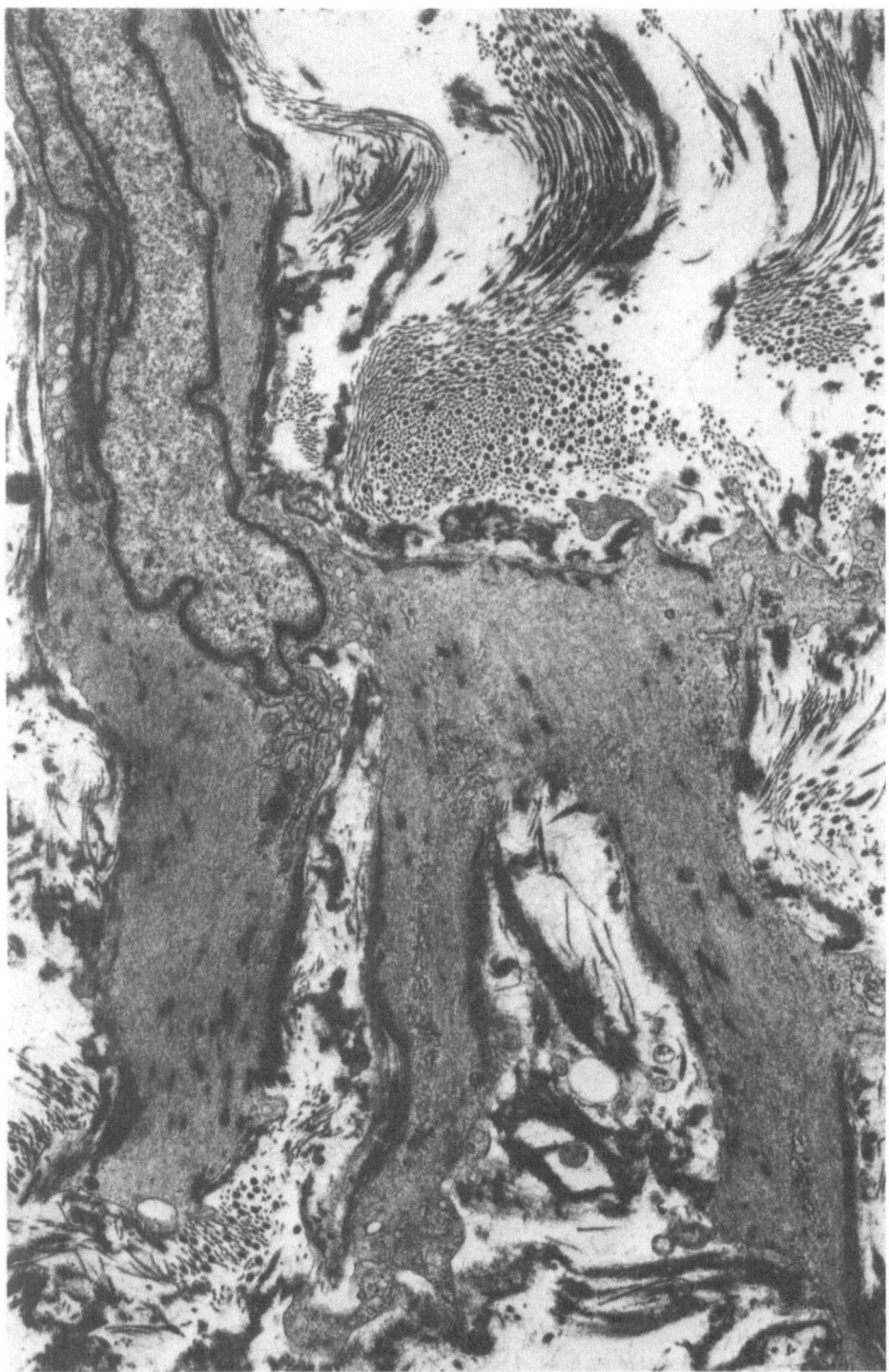

Fig. 1.4. Electron micrograph of an atypical calyceal smooth muscle cell showing several elongated processes extending from the cell body which contains bundles of myofilaments. ($\times 9600$)

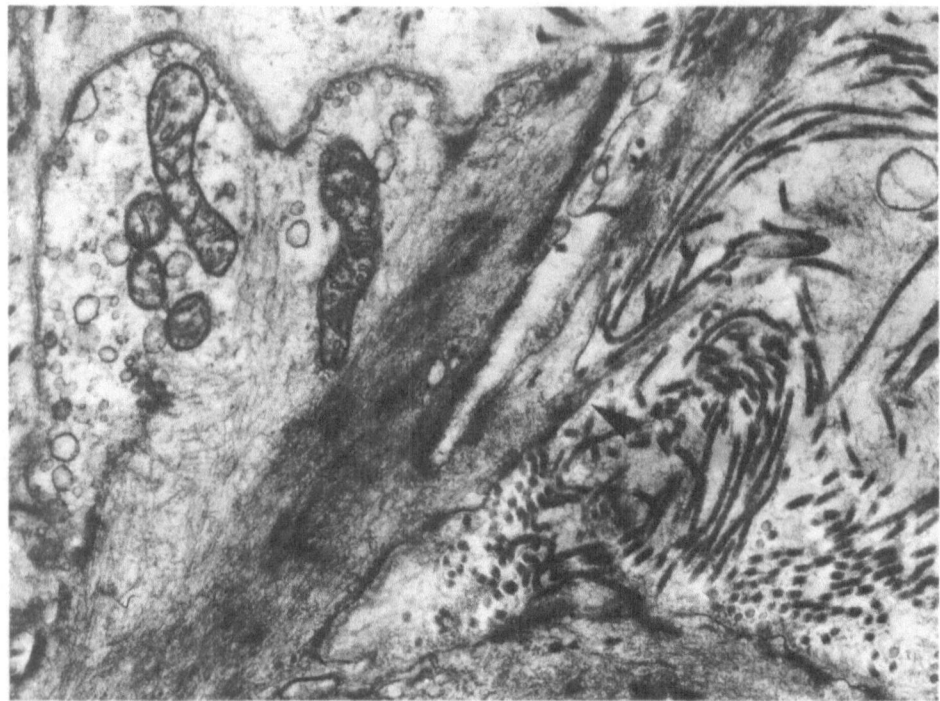

Fig. 1.5. Portion of an atypical cell at higher power. Note the small branch (*arrow*) which lacks surface caveolae and an outer covering of basal lamina. (× 22 400)

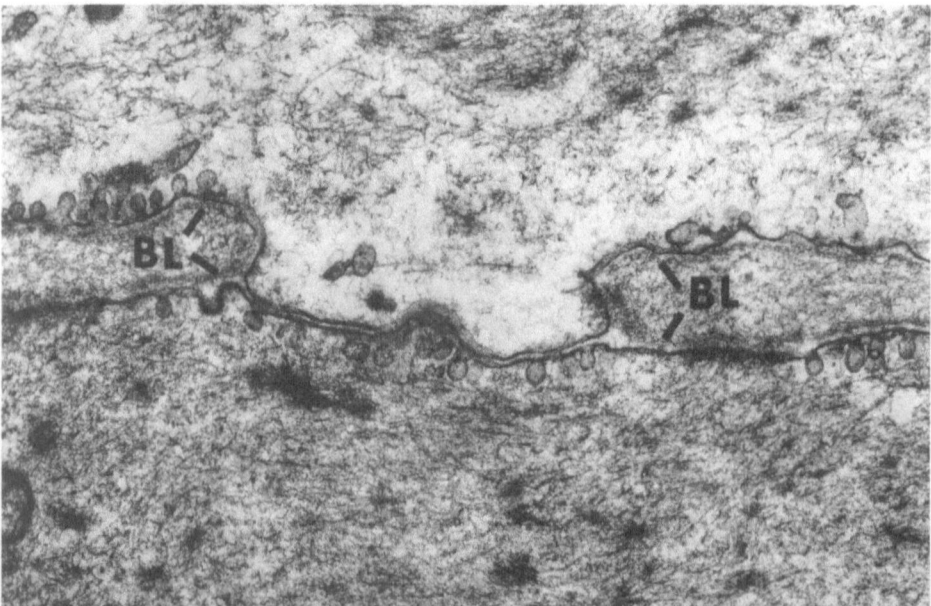

Fig. 1.6. A region of close approach between two smooth muscle cells of the renal pelvic wall. A gap of 20 nm separates the apposing cell membranes while the basal lamina (*BL*) of one cell is reflected at the periphery of the intercellular 'junction' to become continuous with that of its neighbour. (× 31 000)

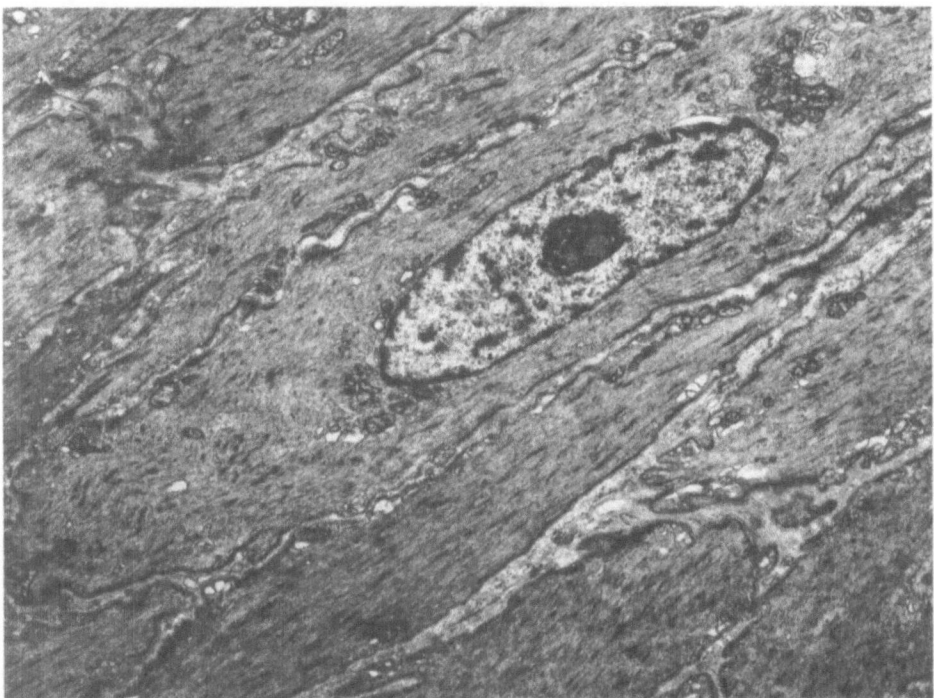

Fig. 1.7. Typical spindle-shaped smooth muscle cells form compact muscle bundles on the outer aspect of the renal pelvic wall. The cells are closely apposed with very little intervening connective tissue and each is packed with myofilaments (cf. Fig. 1.4). (× 6400)

propria. In addition to these perivascular nerves, a few autonomic fibres run independently amongst the smooth muscle bundles. Such nerves are, however, exceedingly sparse when compared with those which innervate the muscle coat of the bladder. Ganglion cells do not occur in the wall of the upper urinary tract.

Functional Considerations

Upper Urinary Tract Contractility

It is well known that under normal conditions contraction waves originate in the proximal part of the upper urinary tract and propagate in an anterograde direction towards the bladder. However, the mechanism involved in the initiation of these contractile events has been the subject of much controversy in the past. One theory proposes that smooth muscle contraction is initiated by the stretching forces exerted by the luminal contents on the muscle coat contained within the walls of the renal calyces and pelvis. However, there is now a considerable body of experimental evidence which demonstrates that the urinary tract possesses spontaneously active regions consisting of pacemaker muscle cells which initiate and exert a controlling influence on the peristaltic activity of the ureter. From a morphological viewpoint, it seems likely that the smooth muscle cells which occur at the attachment of each minor calyx and which are structurally distinct from those elsewhere may act as pacemaker sites. Since each minor calyx possesses such cells (and is linked across the renal parenchyma to other calyces by similar cells), the number of pacemaker sites within a given system is related to the number of minor calyces. It seems probable that the normal sequence of events begins with the initiation of a contraction wave at one of the several minor calyceal pacemaker sites. Once initiated, the contraction is propagated through the wall of the adjacent major calyx and activates the smooth muscle of the renal pelvis. To what extent the inner layer of atypical cells acts as pacemaker (or as a preferential conduction pathway) remains to be determined. The proximal pacemaker site for successive contractions usually changes between the minor calyces, although sometimes the same minor calyx will initiate several consecutive contractions before changing to another minor calyx. Functionally, the proximal location of these pacemaker sites ensures that, once initiated, contraction waves are propagated away from the kidney, thereby avoiding undesirable pressure rises directed against the renal parenchyma. In addition, since several potential pacemaker sites exist, the initiation of contraction waves is unimpaired by partial nephrectomy because the minor calyces spared by the resection remain in situ and continue their pacemaking function.

Each contraction wave extends across the renal pelvis as far as the pelviureteric region, and it seems likely that the onward transmission into the ureter is dependent upon the volume of fluid contained within the renal pelvis. At high urine flow rates, every contraction wave reaching the pelviureteric region is propagated as a ureteral contraction wave. At low flow rates, not all renal pelvic contractions are transmitted into the ureter. Only when a sufficient quantity of urine has accumulated in the renal pelvis does a pelvic contraction wave propagate distally beyond the pelviureteric region. Thus, the pelviureteric region acts as a 'gate', allowing ureteral peristalsis to occur only when the volume of each bolus of urine propelled from the renal pelvis is above a critical amount.

In summary, ureteral peristalsis is apparently dependent upon two mechanisms within the proximal part of the urinary tract. Firstly, contraction waves in the renal pelvis are initiated by spontaneously active pacemaker sites located within the wall of each minor calyx. Secondly, a regulating mechanism at the pelviureteric region determines whether each contraction of the renal pelvis is propagated into the ureter. The latter event is related to urine flow and probably depends upon the stretching forces or tension generated in the wall of the pelviureteric region. It is not yet known whether a malfunction of one or both of these mechanisms is involved in the aetiology of functional obstruction of the upper urinary tract.

Propagation of Peristaltic Contractions

The means by which contraction waves are propagated across the renal pelvis and along the ureter is worthy of further consideration. The most likely mechanism is that of myogenic conduction resulting from electrotonic coupling of one muscle cell to its immediate neighbours. Considerable experimental evidence exists which indicates that autonomic nerves do not play a major part in the propagation of upper urinary tract contraction waves. Firstly, the electrical activity measured in the ureteric wall during peristalsis, together with the rate of propagation of the contraction waves, are characteristic of smooth muscle (and not neural) activity; secondly, the ratio of axons to ureteric smooth muscle cells is extremely low; and thirdly, peristaltic contraction waves not only occur in vivo in the presence of nerve-blocking agents such as tetrodotoxin, but also continue in segments of isolated ureter, which are devoid of functional nervous tissue. Therefore, one must conclude that autonomic nerves are not directly responsible for the propagation of peristaltic waves. The possibility remains, however, that such nerves perform a modulatory role on contractile events which take place within the musculature of the renal calyces, pelvis and ureter.

In several other organs in which myogenic conduction is known to occur, adjacent smooth muscle cells are normally linked by means of the nexus, or gap junction. This specialised region is thought to provide a low resistance pathway allowing electrotonic spread of excitation from one cell to another. It is surprising, therefore, that upper urinary tract smooth muscle is typified by a relative paucity of this type of cell-to-cell contact. However, regions of close approach are extremely numerous between ureteric smooth muscle cells. Thus it seems probable that it is intercellular junctions of this type (rather than gap junctions) which are responsible for the conduction of contraction waves from one ureteric smooth muscle cell to the next. A similar hypothesis has been proposed for the longitudinal muscle coat of the gut wall where the cells are known to be electrically coupled in the absence of gap junctions.

In summary, the contraction waves arising from the upper end of the urinary tract are thought to be propagated from muscle cell to muscle cell by means of intercellular junctions. This process is essentially a property of smooth muscle and does not require the direct involvement of autonomic nerves. The direction of propagation is normally from the renal pelvis towards the bladder, as dictated by the pacemaker mechanism in the minor calyces. Since muscle cells may conduct from one cell to the next in either direction, the direction of propagation may sometimes be reversed resulting in retrograde contraction waves.

Structure of the Upper Urinary Tract in Idiopathic Hydronephrosis

The introduction of radioisotope diuresis renography (see Chap. 4) has enabled the functional capability of the upper urinary tract in suspected cases of idiopathic hydronephrosis to be more accurately assessed (O'Reilly et al. 1978). The technique thus allows greater precision in the selection of patients who are likely to benefit from appropriate surgical treatment— it is on specimens removed from such patients that the following structural analysis is based.

'Dilated' Segment of the Upper Urinary Tract

The majority of specimens from dismembered (Anderson–Hynes) pyeloplasties include a segment of the proximal part of the ureter which, on macroscopic examination, appears to be of normal dimensions. In the pelviureteric region an abrupt increase in diameter occurs (sometimes accompanied by an obvious increase in thickness) and this dilatation involves the whole of the resected renal pelvic wall (together with the calyces in nephrectomy specimens) (Gosling and Dixon 1978).

Histological examination shows that an increase in connective tissue (both collagen and elastic fibres) begins in the junctional region between the non-dilated

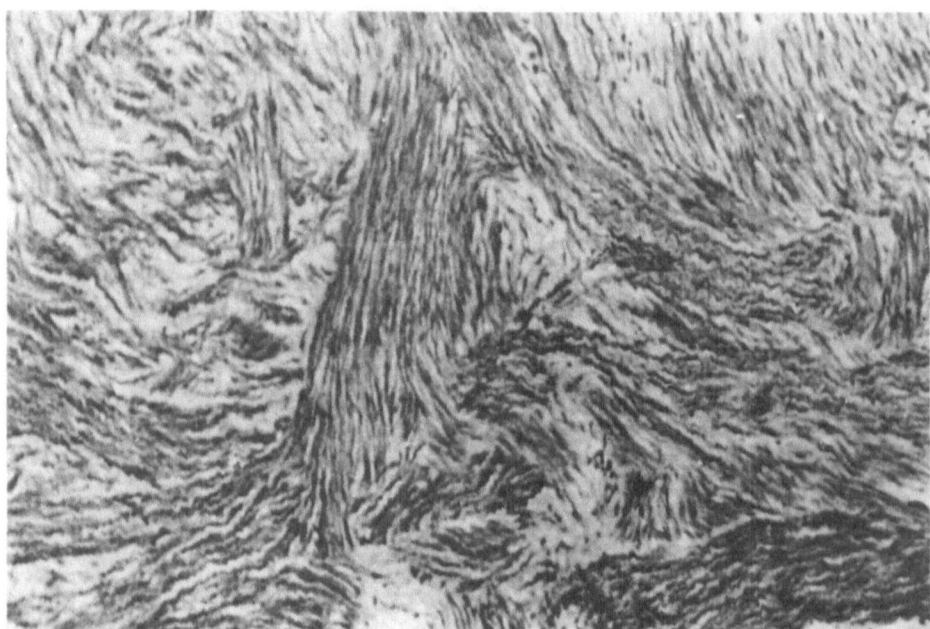

Fig. 1.8. Section through the wall of the renal pelvis from a patient with idiopathic hydronephrosis. Large amounts of connective tissue are present within the muscle bundles such that individual smooth muscle cells are separated from one another. (× 250)

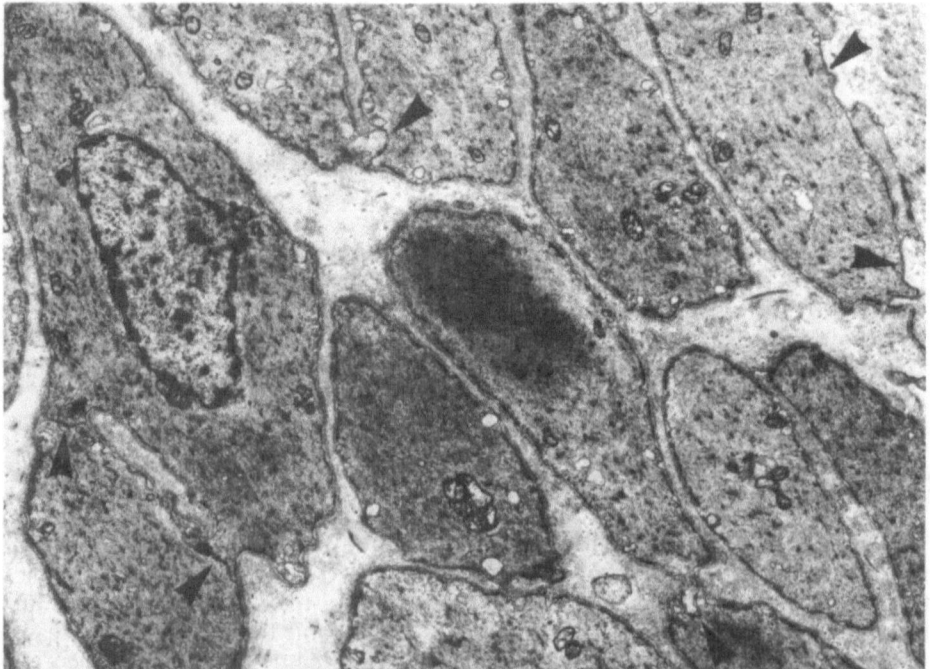

Fig. 1.9. Electron micrograph of smooth muscle cells from a dilated renal pelvis. The increase in intercellular connective tissue is apparent when compared with Fig. 1.7. Regions of close approach between neighbouring muscle cells are still clearly evident (*arrows*). (× 7800)

and dilated segments and extends from this zone throughout the proximal (dilated) part of the urinary tract. This excess connective tissue (Fig. 1.8) is particularly prominent amongst the smooth muscle cells forming the inner aspect of the muscle coat, and usually increases the thickness of the lamina propria. Connective tissue also extends into the muscle bundles forming the outer aspect of the muscle coat, and these elements are seen to separate individual smooth muscle cells from their neighbours. This infiltration occurs throughout all parts of the dilated segment of the urinary tract and is not confined to any particular region.

As noted previously, smooth muscle cells lying in the outer aspect of the normal renal pelvic wall contain large amounts of tissue cholinesterase. In idiopathic hydronephrosis, however, muscle bundles in similar locations are relatively devoid of such enzyme activity. This biochemical deficiency extends throughout the dilated segment and presumably reflects a change in the functional properties of renal pelvic (and calyceal) smooth muscle.

When the electron microscope is used to examine specimens of the hydronephrotic renal pelvis, the smooth muscle cells are seen to be separated from one another by unusually large amounts of connective tissue. The latter consists of bundles of randomly orientated collagen fibres together with numerous pale-staining elastic fibres. Many of these elastic fibres possess dense microfilaments around the periphery, which appear to be in continuity with the basal laminae of adjacent smooth muscle cells. Despite the increased amounts of connective tissue, regions of close approach between adjacent smooth muscle cells are observed with a similar frequency to those in non-dilated ureteric segments (Fig. 1.9).

Marked changes in the fine structure of many of the smooth muscle cells are also evident in most sections from dilated portions of the upper urinary tract. These alterations in fine structure, whilst similar in all samples from the same distended segment, do vary from one specimen to another. In some cases the smooth muscle cells show a considerable increase in their complement of granular reticulum and Golgi membranes, particularly in the perinuclear zone (Fig. 1.10). In these instances the myofilaments are confined to the periphery and some cells also contain numerous membrane-bound dense bodies and lipid droplets. In other specimens many of the smooth muscle cells contain a marked increase in electron-dense bodies which often form clusters within the sarcoplasm.

However, in all cases the most commonly observed fine structural change within the smooth muscle cells consists of a marked decrease in the complement of myofilaments; such cells often display large electron-lucent regions within their sarcoplasm and a reduced number of caveolae. Other cells appear totally devoid of myofilaments and possess pyknotic nuclei, randomly scattered small mitochondria and very few surface caveolae (Fig. 1.11).

'Non-dilated' Segment of the Upper Urinary Tract

Muscle bundles can be traced histologically without interruption from the dilated renal pelvis through the apparently narrow pelviureteric region into the proximal segment of ureter. From the pelviureteric region the arrangement and histochemical properties of ureteric smooth muscle together with the distribution of connective tissue are indistinguishable from control specimens. Also, electron microscopy has shown the structure of the proximal ureter in idiopathic hydronephrosis to be similar to normal material.

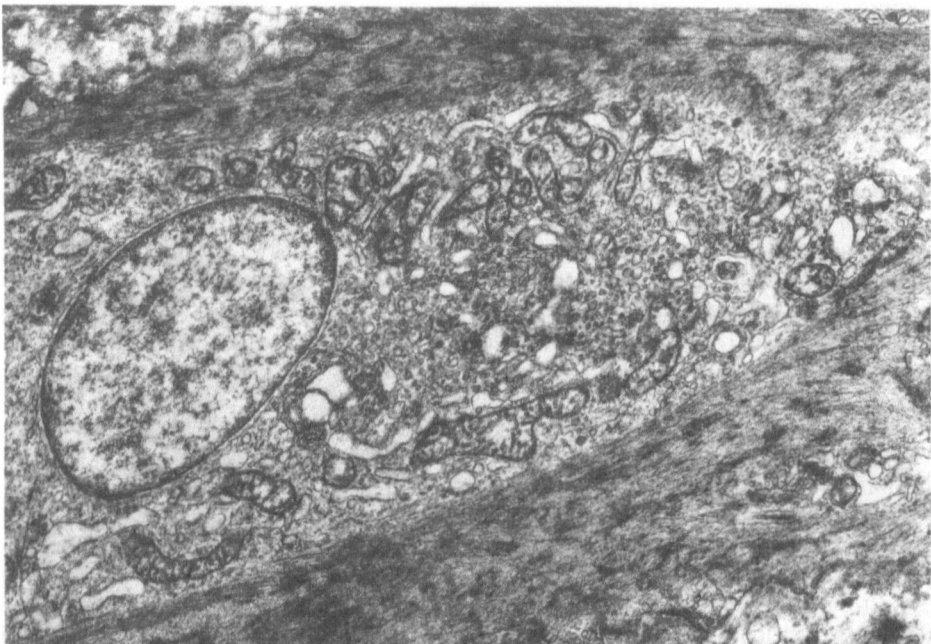

Fig. 1.10. Electron micrograph of a portion of a smooth muscle cell from a case of idiopathic hydronephrosis. The central region of the cell contains extensive granular reticulum, Gogli membranes and mitochondria while the myofilaments are confined to the cell periphery. (×14500)

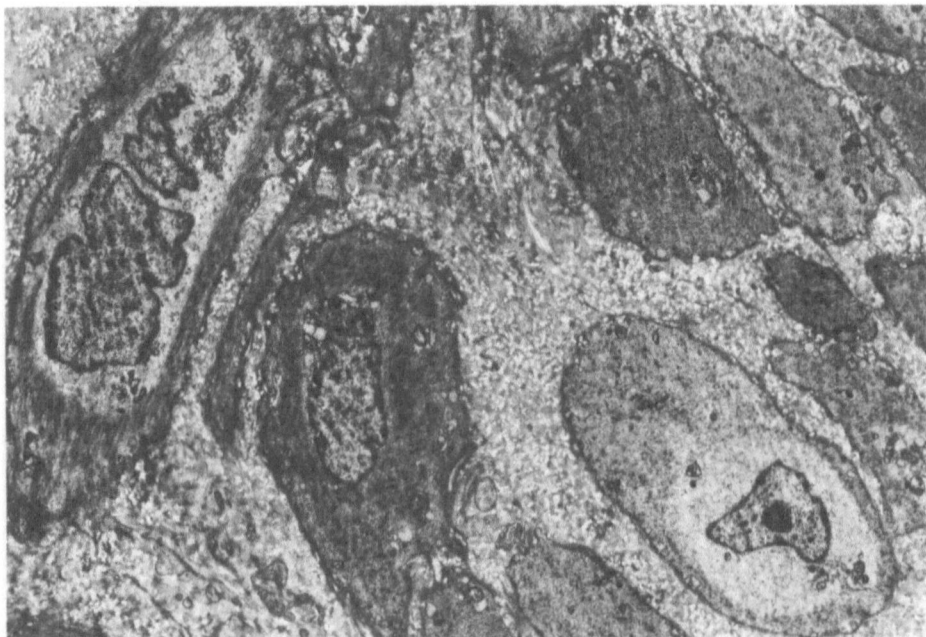

Fig. 1.11. Low power electron micrograph of several smooth muscle cells from a dilated renal pelvic wall. Some of the cells display a marked absence of myofilaments from the perinuclear zone. (×4100)

Aetiological Considerations in Idiopathic Hydronephrosis

The structural changes which have been shown to affect the dilated part of the upper urinary tract in idiopathic hydronephrosis are relevant to previous hypotheses about the basic cause underlying this enigmatic condition. Both Notley (1971, 1972) and Hanna et al. (1976) examined the structure of surgically removed pyeloplasty specimens and proposed that the ureteric segment immediately adjacent to the proximal dilated portion was the part of the urinary tract in which the primary abnormality was to be found. These workers reported a marked increase in collagen, which was confined solely to this particular segment. It was suggested that the connective tissue infiltration formed an inelastic collar which prevented adequate distension of the affected zone during ureteric peristalsis, particularly during diuresis. Although Hanna and co-workers also described morphological changes proximal to this segment, these were thought to arise in response to over-distension and the initial cause was attributed to the collagen-infiltrated 'narrowed' segment of ureter. In contrast, the findings documented in this chapter show that increased amounts of connective tissue do occur but that this excess extends along the entire length of the proximal distended portion of the upper urinary tract. The increase is clearly evident in all cases, including those in which the whole of the proximal distended segment is available for study (viz. nephrectomy specimens). This infiltration of connective tissue extends distally as far as the narrowed segment, where it ceases abruptly. The structure of the so-called narrowed segment of ureter in idiopathic hydronephrosis is indistinguishable both histochemically and fine-structurally from normal preparations. Concerning the obvious conflict between these results and those of earlier workers, it is pertinent to note that both Notley (1968, 1972) and Hanna et al. (1976) did not describe the structure of tissue samples of the distended upper urinary tract which had been obtained at sites remote from the zone of apparent narrowing (i.e., those which can be obtained only from nephrectomy specimens). Furthermore, the results described by these previous authors were based largely upon electron microscopy— a method which invariably limits the size and amount of tissue that can be satisfactorily examined. Thus, the relatively restricted location of the tissue samples together with the limitations of the methods used by these workers may account for the difference between their findings and those presently described. The concept that a narrow segment of ureter causes the condition of idiopathic hydronephrosis is not supported by our own findings.

It is interesting to speculate on the origin of the increased amounts of connective tissue that extend throughout the dilated segment, since there is some evidence to suggest that the smooth muscle cells of this segment may be directly involved in the manufacture of the elastin and collagen. Fine fibrils of elastin extend from the basal laminae of these cells and apparently aggregate into large elastic fibres. In addition, the deposition of numerous collagen fibres separating individual smooth muscle cells occurs in the absence of an increase in the fibroblast component of the smooth muscle coat. In some muscle cells, a marked reduction in the complement of myofilaments is accompanied by an increase in endoplasmic reticulum. Such changes indicate that these cells have increased those organelles which are believed to be involved in active synthesis, seemingly at the expense of their contractile apparatus. Although Notley (1971) and Hanna et al. (1976) failed to comment upon the source of the excessive connective tissue which they observed, the view that smooth muscle is responsible for the manufacture of these components receives support from the work of Ross and Klebanoff (1971) and Gerrity et al. (1975). In this context, the marked difference in tissue cholinesterase between the dilated upper urinary tract and control preparations provides additional evidence of a change in the functional activity of smooth muscle in idiopathic hydronephrosis. It may be that this reduction of enzyme in smooth muscle within the wall of the distended segment is directly related to the manufacture of connective tissue by these cells.

Concerning intercellular relationships, our own studies have substantiated the finding of Notley (1971) and shown that alterations in the fine structure of regions of close approach between adjacent smooth muscle cells do not occur. In addition, the structure and distribution of the nerves which supply the upper urinary tract in cases of idiopathic hydronephrosis are similar to those in control material. Thus, on this evidence, it seems unlikely that the condition is caused by failure of electrotonic coupling between smooth muscle cells or is due to alterations in the autonomic innervation of the upper urinary tract. To what extent the infiltration of connective tissue affects the normal function of either of the two types of smooth muscle (typical and atypical) is not known at present. Finally, consideration should be given as to whether the connective tissue infiltration and altered smooth muscle morphology in idiopathic hydronephrosis represents a primary or a secondary response. Indirect evidence in support of the latter possibility has recently been obtained from investigation of the mechanically obstructed lower urinary tract (Gosling and Dixon 1980). In patients in whom bladder outflow obstruction has induced trabeculation and ureteric reflux, connective tissue infiltration and altered smooth muscle morphology of the type seen in idiopathic hydronephrosis also occurs in both the bladder and ureters. In addition, Gee and Kiviat (1975) reported an increase in connective tissue together with alterations in the fine structure of smooth muscle in the proximal urinary tract of the rabbit, which they were able to produce by partially obstructing the ureter. Hence, the muscle coat responds to mechanical obstruction by secondarily increasing the connective tissue components within the wall of the urinary tract. Furthermore, the data presented in Chap. 2 show that the contractile behaviour of the upper urinary tract in idiopathic hydronephrosis is indistinguishable from that of the distended renal pelvis produced experimentally by mechanically obstructing the ureter.

To conclude, the morphological changes seen in the upper urinary tract in idiopathic hydronephrosis, which occur as a secondary consequence of an unknown functional obstruction, are of value in assessing the degree to which this obstruction has progressed. However, only when the cause for this obstruction has been resolved will the aetiology of idiopathic hydronephrosis be fully understood.

References

Gee WF, Kiviat MD (1975) Ureteral response to partial obstruction. Invest Urol 12: 309–316

Gerrity RG, Adams EP, Cliff WJ (1975) The aortic tunica media of the developing rat. II. Incorporation by medial cells of ^{3}H-proline into collagen and elastin. Autoradiographic and chemical studies. Lab Invest 32: 601–609

Gosling JA, Dixon JS (1978) Functional obstruction of the ureter and renal pelvis. A histological and electron microscopic study. Br J Urol 50: 145–152

Gosling JA, Dixon JS (1980) Structure of trabeculated detrusor smooth muscle in cases of prostatic hypertrophy. Urol Int 35: 351–355

Hanna MK, Jeffs RD, Sturgess JM, Barkin M (1976) Ureteral structure and ultrastructure. II. Congenital ureteropelvic junction obstruction and primary obstructive megaureter. J Urol 116: 725–730

Notley RG (1968) Electron microscopy of the upper ureter and the pelvi-ureteric junction. Br J Urol 40: 37–52

Notley RG (1971) The structural basis for normal and abnormal ureteric motility. Ann R Coll Surg Engl 49: 250–267

Notley RG (1972) Electron microscopy of the primary obstructive megaureter. Br J Urol 44: 229–234

O'Reilly PH, Testa HJ, Lawson RS, Farrar DJ, Charlton-Edwards E (1978) Diuresis renography in equivocal urinary tract obstruction. Br J Urol 50: 76–80

Ross R, Klebanoff SJ (1971) The smooth muscle cell. I. In vivo synthesis of connective tissue proteins. J Cell Biol 50: 159–171

2. Urodynamics of the Multicalyceal Upper Urinary Tract

C.E. Constantinou and J.C. Djurhuus

The upper urinary tract consists of the calyces, renal pelvis and ureters, all of which are involved in the active transport of urine away from the kidney towards the bladder. Clearly, before the mechanism of urine transport in this system can be understood, the contribution made by each of the component parts must be defined.

In this chapter our current knowledge of the properties of each segment is considered and discussed. Data will be presented from physiological studies carried out on the porcine multicalyceal kidney in vivo and in vitro. A section is included dealing with the regulating mechanisms of urine transport in the intact upper urinary tract. In addition, the effects of experimental ureteric obstruction upon this system are considered. In outline the chapter deals in turn with (a) the frequency of contraction of individual calyces, (b) the relationship between calyceal frequency and fluid flow rate, (c) coupling between calyces and renal pelvis, (d) coupling between renal pelvis and the ureter, (e) the hydrodynamics of renal pelvic filling and emptying, (f) regulation of bolus volume and peristaltic rate by urine flow rate, and (g) the effects of experimental obstruction on the regulation of bolus volume and peristaltic rate, and conduction of renal pelvic contractions. Finally, parameters are considered in the light of clinical observations made on cases of idiopathic hydronephrosis. Previously published reports of clinical and experimental studies on the upper urinary tract have been ably reviewed by Weiss (1976, 1979) and recent data obtained from multicalyceal systems are presented elsewhere in the present volume.

Functional Activity of the Normal Upper Urinary Tract

In dealing with the characterisation of calyceal and renal pelvic activity an experimental model has been used in an effort to minimise movement artefacts produced by respiration. For this purpose, porcine kidneys have been surgically removed and perfused to enable recordings to be made from individual calyces over extended periods of time. Fine fluid-filled pressure sensors passed through the calyceal system have been used to record the contractile force generated by individual calyces. In this system the sensor is located in the region of the papillae so as to record pressure generated in the adjacent calyceal wall. Connections to the recording system are made by passing a fluid-filled system through the renal parenchyma. In this experimental model the attachment of the calyces are not disturbed by the recording apparatus and simultaneous measurements from several calyces can be obtained. A typical recording from four calyces is shown in Fig. 2.1. The amplitude and phase of the hydrostatic pressure from the upper, middle, and lower regions of the calyceal system are recorded. Some measurements provide experimental evidence to show that the calyces undergo continuous rhythmical

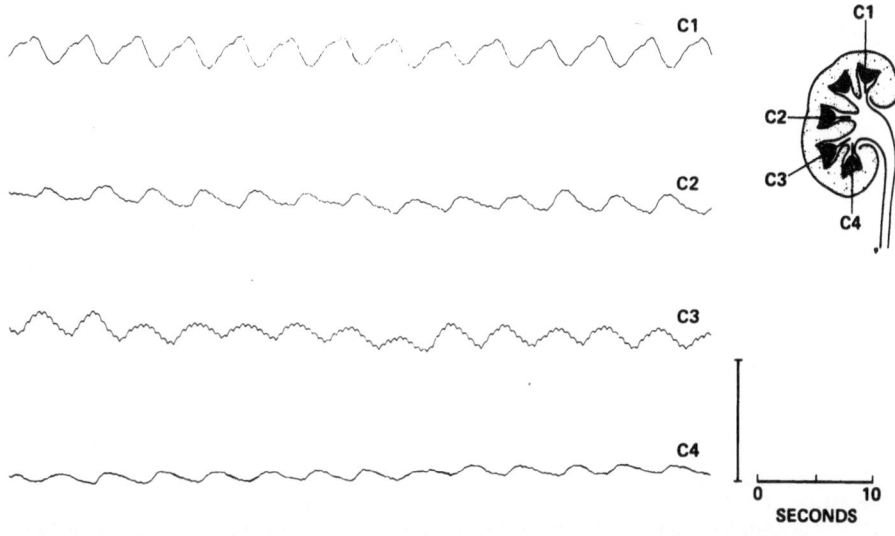

Fig. 2.1. Regular spontaneous contractility in four calyces. Simultaneous pressure measurements made on the perfused kidney. The frequency of contraction of each calyx is similar to that of the other calyces. Although the onset of individual contractile events are not synchronous with those of the adjoining calyces, the phase angle between calyces remains relatively constant. The diagram *inset* identifies the placement of pressure detection sensors (*C1–C4*). The waveform obtained by each pressure sensor is correspondingly identified. *Vertical scale,* 20 cmH$_2$O.

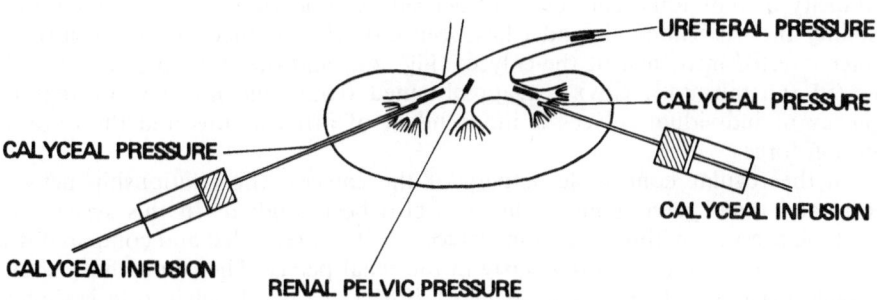

Fig. 2.2. Diagrammatic representation of experimental model used for the infusion at varying flow rates of individual calyces. As shown, infusion is through a catheter lying parallel to the pressure sensing probe. Variations in the calyceal flow rate are effected by changing the infusion rate of the pumping mechanism.

contractions with a frequency of 12/min. The amplitude of these contractions is 3–5 cmH$_2$O and are sinusoidal in wave form. The presence of rhythmical calyceal contractions in the absence of distension or neuronal input supports the view that calyceal smooth muscle is capable of contracting spontaneously. Interestingly, there is no significant variation in calyceal frequency between those located either in the upper or lower poles of the kidney. In addition, the phase between the onset of

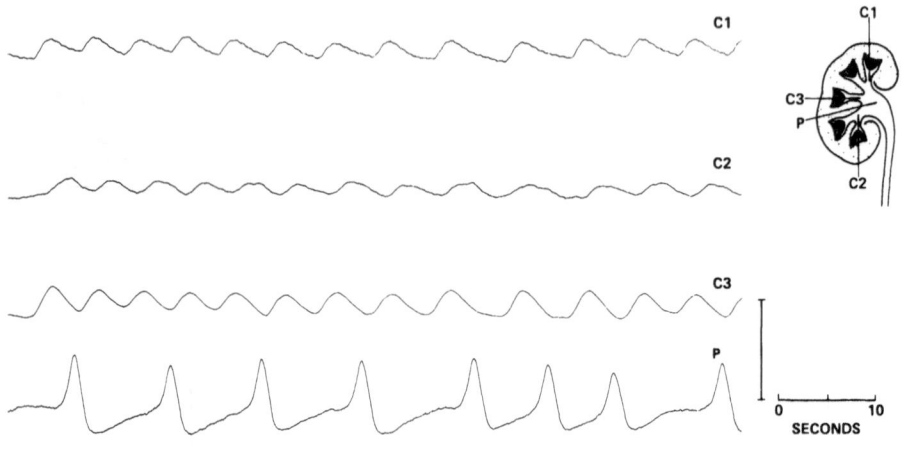

Fig. 2.3. Comparison between calyceal and renal pelvic contractility. As shown schematically in the *inset*, in three calyces, *C1-C3*, pressure oscillations are recorded simultaneously together with renal pelvic pressure *P*. The corresponding waveforms from each sensor are indicated. *Vertical scale,* 20 cmH$_2$O.

calyceal contractions remains constant over relatively long periods of time, indicating a degree of synchronisation. Finally, the frequency of small isolated calyceal segments studied in vitro has shown autorhythmicity to be an inherent property of calyceal tissue and is independent of structural continuity with other parts of the upper urinary tract.

Based upon the observation that the calyceal system contracts rhythmically in the absence of external stimuli, the question naturally arises as to whether the rhythmicity of individual calyces is influenced by fluid flow rate. To explore this possibility the experimental model has been modified to incorporate an infusion catheter inserted into each of the calyces (Fig. 2.2) and the flow rate varied in the range 0.1-0.6 ml.min^{-1}. calyx^{-1}. Data obtained from this model show that the frequency of individual calyces is independent of infused flow and the resulting distension forces.

Given the regular contractile activity of the calyces, the relationship between calyceal and renal pelvic contractility has also been studied. In this system, the hydrostatic pressure within individual calyces has been recorded and compared with the pressure monitored simultaneously in the renal pelvis. The results have shown that while calyceal rate is independent of flow rate, renal pelvic rate is directly related to fluid flow. Figure 2.3 illustrates the characteristic waveforms of pressures within three calyces and the renal pelvis. Based upon an analysis of results similar to those illustrated in Fig. 2.3, calyceal contractions are in phase with each other and with the contractions occurring in the wall of the renal pelvis. The difference in frequency between the calyces and the renal pelvis appears to be an inherent property of the cellular organisation of these structures. Evidence relating to the inherent frequency of the calyceal and renal pelvic preparations has been provided by isolating small tissue strips and monitoring the frequency of spontaneous contractions from each region. Figure 2.4 illustrates the asymmetric contractions recorded from the two individual calyceal strips and two renal pelvic strips. The renal pelvic strips undergo tension changes which occur at a rate approximately similar to that of renal pelvic contraction in the intact preparation (10-12/min).

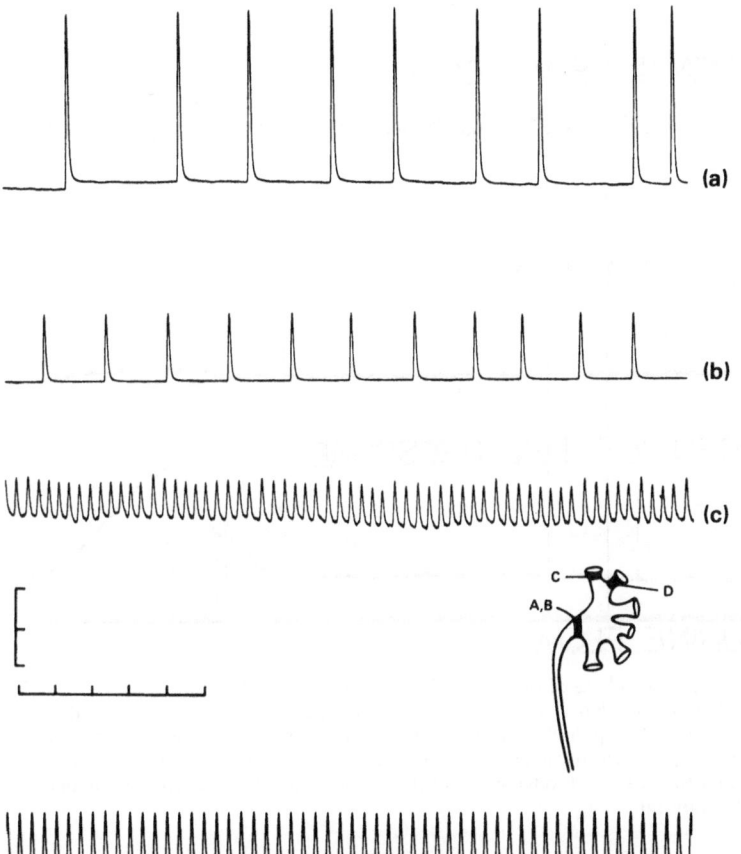

Fig. 2.4. Autorhythmicity of renal pelvic and calyceal muscle strips in vitro. The contractile rate of renal pelvic strips (**a, b**) shows a broad frequency spectrum, which is dependent upon anatomical position. Conversely, it is shown that calyceal contraction rate (**c, d**) has a higher frequency of contraction and a narrow spectrum. *Horizontal scale* is calibrated in 30-s intervals; *vertical scale* in grams.

Renal pelvic strips exhibit tension changes, the rate of which depends upon position. Thus, proximal regions show isometric contractions at a rate of 5–6/min; distal strips contract at lower rates.

Combined measurements of calyceal and renal pelvic pressures have shown that the rate of contractions of the renal pelvis is, under most circumstances, significantly lower than that of the calyces. However, the integration between calyceal and renal pelvic contractions is suggestive of a mechanism whereby the calyces initiate activity in the wall of the renal pelvis. Since a rise in the pelvic pressure does not produce a concomitant pressure rise in the calyces, it is concluded that the latter are isolated hydrodynamically from the expulsive pressures of the pelvis. Consideration of the spontaneous rhythmicity of tissue segments removed from the pelvicalyceal junction suggests that an abrupt change in the frequency of spontaneous activity occurs. As previously noted, the frequency of spontaneous contractions falls from the renal pelvis, indicating a frequency gradient.

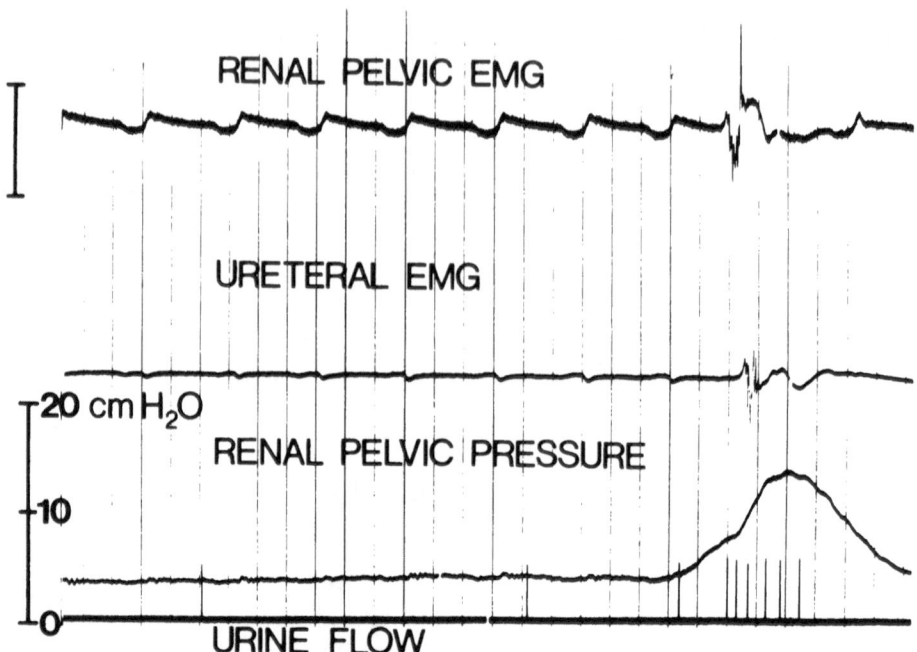

Fig. 2.5. Illustration of the filling phase of the renal pelvis at a mean urine flow rate of approximately 0.2 ml.min^{-1} ureter^{-1}. It is shown that at this flow rate the renal pelvic pressure remains at the low pressure of ~3 cmH$_2$O over a 30-s period. The onset of a systolic contraction elevates renal pelvic pressure to 12 cmH$_2$O. Renal pelvic electrical activity is detected approximately 2 s after the onset of the contraction, indicating that the origin is located distal to the region in which the electrodes are placed. Time lines are of 1-s repetition rate.

Anaesthetised pigs have been used to record the electrical activity of the renal pelvis and ureter over a broad range of diuretic conditions, and these measurements have been supplemented by pressure recordings from within the renal pelvis. The volume of the bolus accompanying each contraction has also been determined by means of ureteric catheterisation procedures. These studies have provided data on the propagation characteristics of the upper urinary tract.

Figure 2.5 shows the sequence of events which occur in association with a renal pelvic and ureteric contraction. The renal pelvic pressure wave can be divided into four stages: (1) filling stage, during which the renal pelvis accumulates urine delivered from the calyces, (2) renal pelvic contraction associated with bolus formation, (3) bolus expulsion, and finally (4) ureteric peristalsis. In the filling stage, renal pelvic pressure is maintained at approximately 2–5 cmH$_2$O. The filling stage terminates with the onset of a renal pelvic contraction and an increase in pressure to approximately 12 cmH$_2$O. This contraction, which is accompanied by an action potential, is propagated throughout the length of the ureter without interruption.

In separating the filling phase from the emptying phase of the renal pelvis it is better to study the behaviour of the pelvis and the ureter during the transition from low to high fluid flow.

Analysis of a typical experiment is presented in Fig. 2.6, where interperistaltic interval and bolus volume have been plotted during a 60-min period. It is evident

EFFECT OF DIURESIS ON PERISTALSIS AND
BOLUS VOLUME ON INTACT KIDNEY

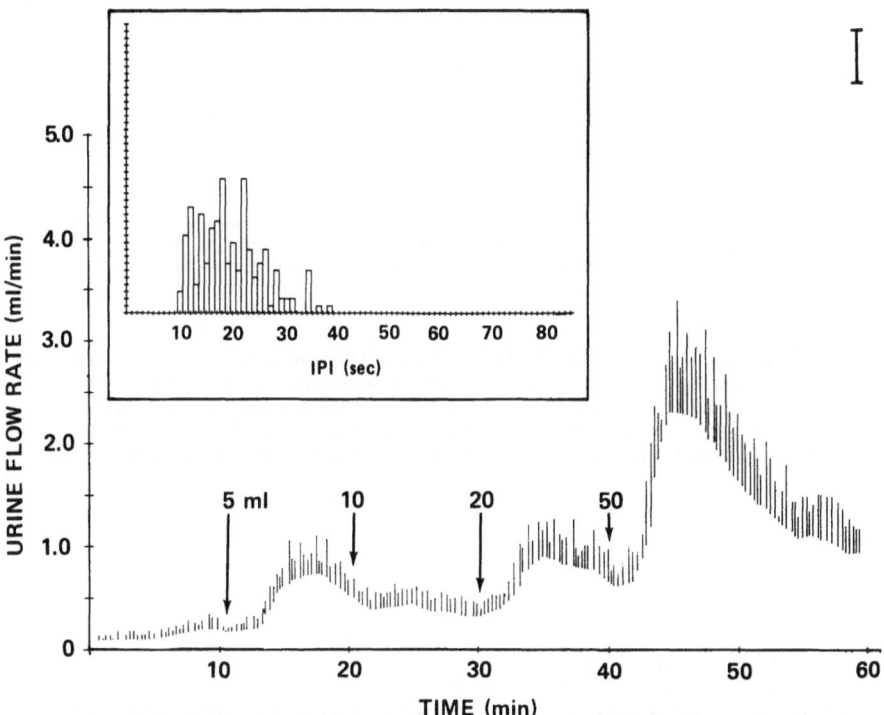

Fig. 2.6. Temporal and distributive properties of ureteral peristaltic rate and bolus volume from a 60-min period of measurement. *Spacing* between the *vertical lines* represents the duration of the interperistaltic intervals; their *length,* the volume of the urine bolus. The calibration for 1.0 ml bolus is shown on the *upper right* of the illustration. The *vertical line* represents the running mean of urine flow rate with a 60-s window. Calibration of urine flow rate is indicated on the *vertical axis. Arrows* indicate intravenous injections of mannitol stimulating diuresis at increasingly higher levels. The volume of mannitol administered is also shown. *Inset* represents a histogram of interperistaltic intervals (IPI) of all data obtained in this preparation.

that while urine flow rate increases from 0.1 ml/min to over 2.5 ml/min, ureteric peristaltic rate changes from 1.5/min to 6/min. This maximum rate is attained during the time when the flow rate increase is highest. Rapid alterations in the rate of urine flow which occur during the administration of a diuretic bolus are accommodated by an increase both in bolus volume and peristaltic rate. Saturation of peristaltic rate results in a slight elevation of the resting renal pelvic pressure and an increase in the amplitude of contraction pressure, as demonstrated in Fig. 2.7. It is evident from this illustration that electrical events initiated at the renal pelvis are conducted to the ureter in association with a fluid bolus. Regulation of ureteral contraction rate can be studied during the increase of peristalsis which is induced by a stimulus administered at the time of low urine flow. As indicated in Fig. 2.8, the filling renal pelvic pressure remains low (approximately 5 cmH$_2$O) and ureteral peristalsis is triggered at a rate which is seemingly independent of the flow produced. Thus, despite a ten-fold increase in urine flow, the time interval between ureteric

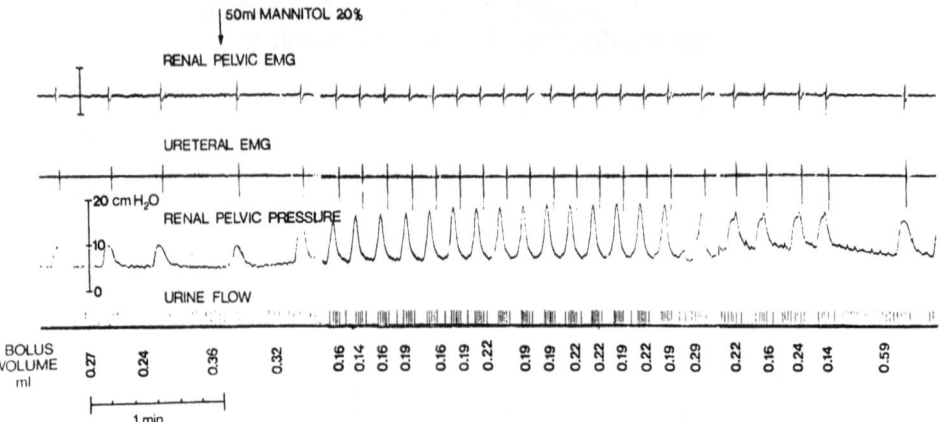

Fig. 2.7. Recording illustrating the effect of a 50-ml mannitol (20%) diuretic stimulus on renal pelvic EMG, ureteric EMG, renal pelvic pressure and bolus volume. The origin of a peristaltic contraction is represented as a systolic pressure rise in the renal pelvis from a baseline pressure of 5 cmH$_2$O. This increase in pressure is associated with electrical activity of the renal pelvis. This electrical activity is propagated to the ureter transporting a urine bolus. The magnitude of each bolus is shown in millimeters.

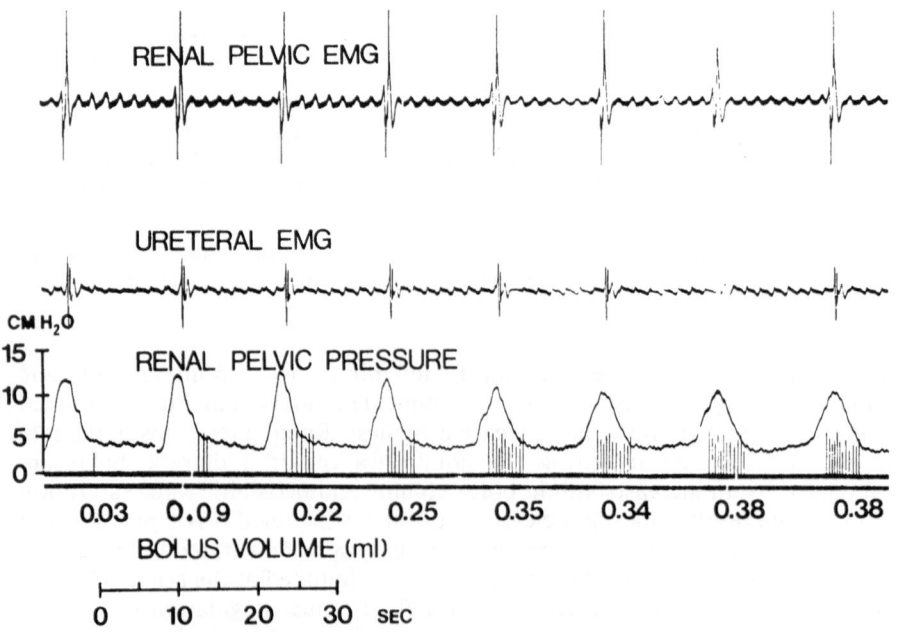

Fig. 2.8. Recording to illustrate that the rate of peristalsis is not dependent upon the bolus under conditions of transient diuresis. Bolus volumes of 0.03–0.38 ml are generated in the renal pelvis and ureter, with insignificant elevation in resting renal pelvic pressure. This figure demonstrates that the onset of peristalsis under conditions where the renal pelvis is at the maximum frequency is a triggered phenomenon and does not directly depend upon the rate of renal pelvic filling or pressure.

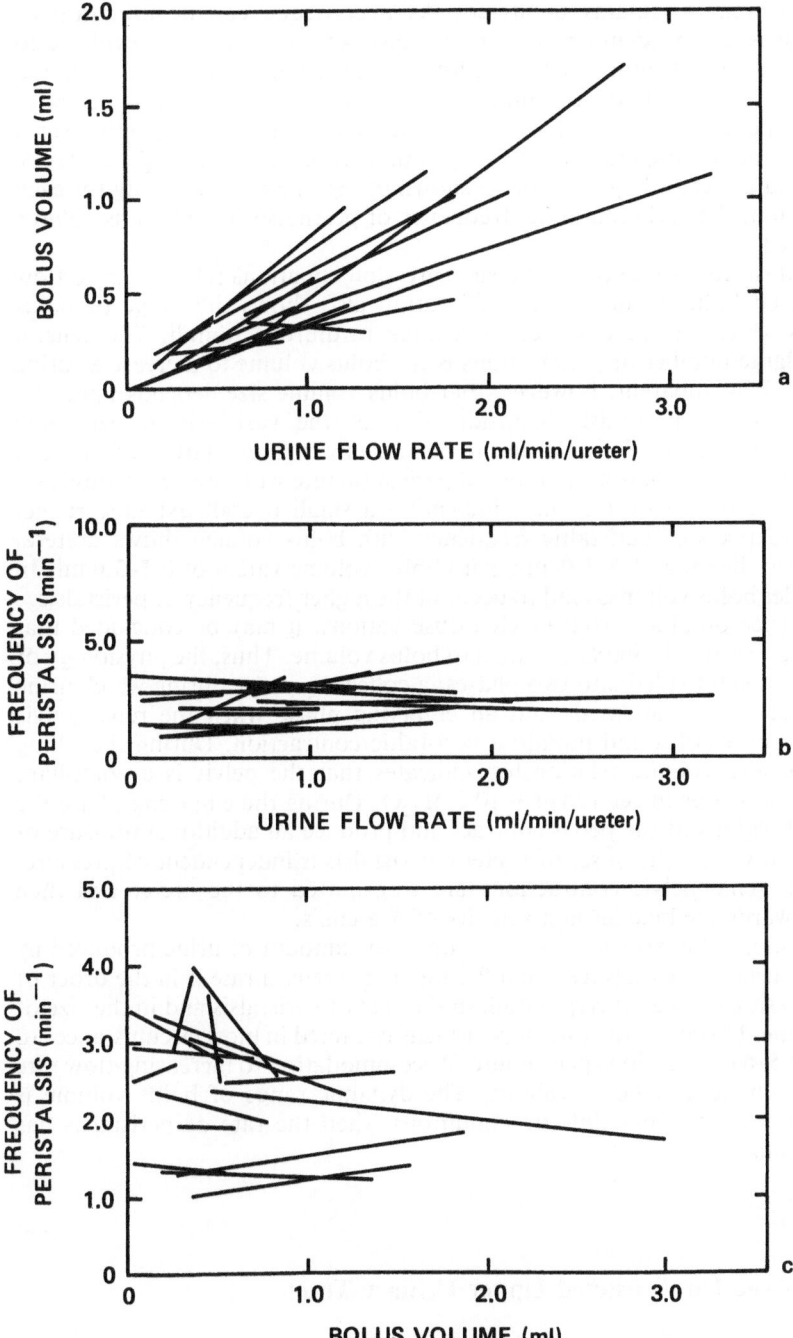

Fig. 2.9. **a** Relationship between bolus volume and urine flow rate in the normal system. Each *line* indicates a regression equation obtained over the range of urine flow rates produced by diuretic stimuli. **b** Relationship between peristaltic frequency and urine flow rate in the normal system. *Lines* represent regression equations for the same range of values shown in **a**. **c** Variation of peristaltic rate and bolus volume in the same preparations as in **a** and **b**.

peristaltic contractions remains unaltered. As a consequence, the initiation of ureteric peristalsis is dependent upon the renal pelvis and, *ipso facto,* is regulated to a maximum rate of 5-6/min. Consideration of the dynamic range of variation between peristaltic rate and bolus volume has been achieved by computing the mean values of each parameter over a fixed period of time. Controlled diuresis over a period of one hour can therefore produce dynamic data characterising the response of the pelvis and ureter. Using the scheme shown in Fig. 2.6 and averaging for each ten minute period, the variation in the frequency of peristalsis and in bolus volume can be evaluated.

Figure 2.9 illustrates a number of linear regression equations relating urine flow rate to measured bolus volume. This illustration also shows the range of bolus volume values which can be obtained in relation to diuretic stimuli. The general tendency in a large number of preparations is for bolus volume to increase as urine flow increases. It is apparent, however, that bolus volume size depends upon the frequency of ureteric peristalsis. Consideration of the variation of peristaltic frequency with respect to bolus volume can be made by further analysis of the data shown in Fig. 2.9. The variations in ureteral peristaltic rate with respect to flow rate are limited in the region of 1-5/min, indicating a small overall dynamic range. Similarly, comparison of peristaltic frequency with bolus volume shows ureteral peristaltic rate in the range 1.5-3.0/min with bolus volume values of 0.1-3.0 ml. In addition, smaller bolus volumes tend to occur at the higher frequency of peristalsis.

On the evidence obtained from in vivo observations, it may be concluded that ureteral peristaltic rate is intimately related to bolus volume. Thus, the physiology of the renal pelvis is subdivided into two phases: a collecting phase during which urine from the calyces is accumulated, and an emptying phase when the renal pelvis contracts to form a bolus and initiate a peristaltic contraction. During the filling phase, the pressure/volume relationship indicates that the pelvis is a compliant system having pressures in the range 3-10 cmH$_2$O. During the emptying phase the most proximal regions of the pelvis contract and produce an additional pressure of 5-10 cmH$_2$O. However, the onset of ureteric peristalsis is independent of pressure. Once initiated, renal pelvic contractions are transmitted to the ureter and then propagated towards the bladder at a velocity of 3-5 cm/s.

The rate of ureteral contraction depends upon the amount of urine produced by the kidney. At urine flow rates less than 0.2 ml/min, ureteral rate is in the order of 2-3/min. Diuresis causes an increase both in the rate of peristalsis and in the size of the bolus volume. However, the rate of peristalsis is limited in most circumstances to a maximum of 5-6 contractions per minute. Accommodation to increasing flow rate is achieved by changes in bolus volume. The dynamic range of bolus volume is particularly important under diuretic conditions when the rate of peristalsis has reached maximum.

Physiology of the Unobstructed Upper Urinary Tract

The results obtained from the unobstructed upper urinary tract have shown that ureteric peristalsis in the multicalyceal system is controlled by the proximal part of the system. Once initiated, pelvic contractions are propagated along the ureter at a rate dependent upon urine flow. Thus, at low levels of diuresis, the pelvis accumulates urine over comparatively long periods of time before the conditions of calyceal renal pelvic coupling are appropriate for the initiation and formation of a bolus and the propagation of a peristaltic contraction. During this collecting phase, pelvic pressure is comparatively low (< 5 cmH$_2$O). On contraction the pelvic pressure increases to reach a maximum of approximately 10 cmH$_2$O. The onset of renal pelvic contractions is initiated from levels that are anatomically higher than the position of the exposed renal pelvis. The mechanism of renal pelvic contraction initiation in the multicalyceal kidney differs from the unicalyceal system (Constantinou 1974). In the unicalyceal kidney of the dog, for example, renal pelvic contractions are conducted by the ureter selectively only under specific conditions of diuresis. As the capacity of the renal pelvis in the multicalyceal kidney is larger than in the unicalyceal kidney, the size of the bolus volume is proportionately larger. The data provided by this study show that the primary determinant in the regulation of urine transport in the multicalyceal kidney is bolus volume. In this sense, the dynamic range of bolus volume is over 30 times that of the dynamic range of the rate of peristalsis. The restriction in the dynamic range of peristaltic rate appers to be due to its inherent limitation in attaining values greater than a given maximum frequency.

Under conditions in which urine flow rate is increased from relatively low to high levels by means of diuretic stimuli, the rate of peristalsis reaches a frequency of approximately 6/min. At maximum frequency further increases of urine flow are accommodated by an increase in the bolus volume. More significantly, these observations indicate that the generation of a urine bolus does not depend upon filling and distension of the renal pelvis. Instead, it can be considered to be a triggered phenomenon with closely regulated limits. Primary supporting evidence substantiating the upper limit of triggering frequency is provided by the fact that the frequency of pelvic contraction becomes constant during rapidly increasing diuresis. These findings provide support for the concept of a calyceal pacemaker system which is responsible for initiating renal pelvic contractions. Anatomical evidence for such a pacemaker system in the multicalyceal kidney has been described in Chap. 1. In this context, in vitro studies have shown that the initiation of coordinated renal pelvic contractions is independent of distension forces (Gosling and Constantinou 1976), and that spontaneous contractility occurs without attachment to other structures such as the calyces.

An alternative theory has proposed that the upper urinary tract is a bi-stable system responding directly to stretch in the absence of an active pacemaker system. In this hypothesis, ureteral contractions occur in response to the accumulation of fluid within the renal pelvis. In such a system it would be expected that the bolus volume remains relatively constant and that increased fluid flow during diuresis would be accommodated by peristaltic rate. As is seen from the foregoing, the available evidence does not support this hypothesis. Furthermore, data relating frequency of peristalsis with urine flow failed to support this alternative concept that a bi-stable system inherently possesses. The wide variation in bolus volume associated with a narrow variation in peristaltic rate is thus evidence against direct muscle stretch as this stimulus to peristalsis.

In summary, urine transport in the upper urinary tract appears to be regulated by a system of pacemakers. These pacemakers are organised in a hierarchical sequence such that the highest inherent frequency occurs within the calyceal system. In the renal pelvis a gradient exists, with the result that the highest frequency regions are those located in the proximal regions of the pelvis. On the basis of the evidence to be presented, obstruction and the ensuing hydronephrosis alter the hierarchical order of pacemaker function in the upper urinary tract. Such disruption causes discoordination of pelvic contractility leading towards incomplete emptying of the contents of the pelvis. Thus residual pelvic urine contributes further towards dilation of the upper urinary tract.

Finally, the organisation of spontaneous contractility within the renal pelvis suggests the possibility of a spatially distributed pacemaker system with regions possessing inherently high frequency of contractions located in the proximal regions and a gradient of increasingly low frequency distally. Such a system has been shown in the unicalyceal kidney (Constantinou et al. 1978; Hannapel and Lutzeyer 1978).

The Experimentally Obstructed Upper Urinary Tract

It has been shown in the preceding section of this chapter that the mechanism determining ureteral peristaltic rate is closely inter-related with bolus volume. Obstruction of the ureter is accompanied by alterations in the geometrical configuration of both the renal pelvis and the ureter. An effort to provide more information on the significance of this distortion is pertinent to define the effects of obstruction upon the regulatory mechanism of urine transport. An experimental in vivo model of hydronephrosis was used for this purpose. With this technique specimens obtained from chronically obstructed preparations demonstrate arrhythmic contractility of both calyceal and renal pelvic structures. Figure 2.10 illustrates a recording obtained from a chronically obstructed preparation. In such preparations it is frequently observed that ureteral peristalsis occurs in bursts of activity. Based upon observations made on the calyceal system, it is apparent that the bursting mode of activity observed in the pelvis originates from the calyceal system. It is apparent from Fig. 2.10 that absence of calyceal contractions results in the absence of renal pelvic contractions. However, the occurrence of calyceal contractions does not necessarly precede renal pelvic activity. It is also apparent from this illustration that both the onset and the cessation of calyceal activity occurs in a coordinated and apparently synchronised manner. Such observations indicate the possible presence of a synchronisation mechanism between the calyces which

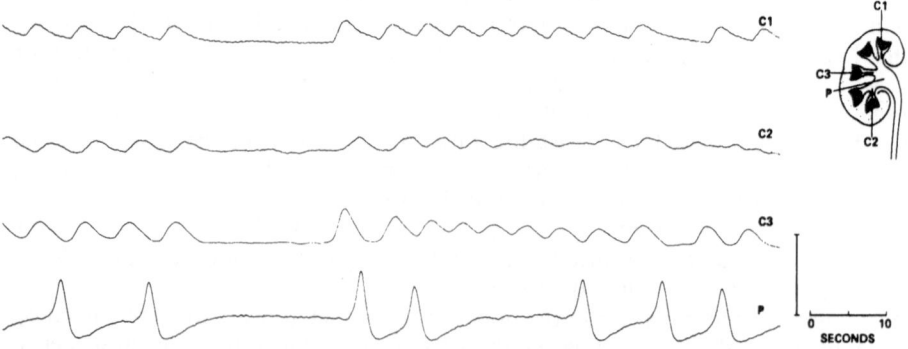

Fig. 2.10. Burst of calyceal and renal pelvic activity in the obstructed system. The pressure sensor placement is indicated on the *inset*. This recording illustrates that the onset of a burst of calyceal activity occurs simultaneously in all measured calyces. It is also shown that activity in the renal pelvis is initiated in phase with the calyces and ends with the cessation of calyceal activity. *Vertical scale*, 20 cmH$_2$O.

Table 2.1. Percent response of urine flow rate, bolus volume, and peristaltic rate to increments of diuretic stimuli in the control and hydronephrotic kidney

Diuretic stimulus	Urine flow rate		Bolus volume	
	Control	Hydronephrotic	Control	Hydronephrotic
5 ml Mannitol 20%	148.3 ± 443.7	21.15 ± 075.0	118.2 ± 372.8	15.8 ± 61.9
10 ml Mannitol 20%	451.8 ± 1082.2	166.90 ± 380.7	449.8 ± 1347.4	61.6 ± 100.9
20 ml Mannitol 20%	779.3 ± 1734.2	199.20 ± 251.7	870.8 ± 2155.1	139.9 ± 234.2
50 ml Mannitol 20%	1243.2 ± 2726.6	637.20 ± 693.9	1229.6± 3017.0	414.2 ± 517.6
10-min Control	1154.3 ± 2475.9	527.30 ± 772.3	1115.7 ± 2418.5	410.0 ± 711.7
20-min Control	975.9 ± 1994.0	416.40 ± 638.6	1080.9 ± 2433.9	388.6 ± 694.4

Table 2.1. (*continued*)

Diuretic stimulus	Peristaltic rate	
	Control	Hydronephrotic
5 ml Mannitol 20%	15.8 ± 24.7	9.7 ± 10.3
10 ml Mannitol 20%	9.4 ± 32.4	19.3 ± 29.6
20 ml Mannitol 20%	12.5 ± 40.8	23.5 ± 30.2
50 ml Mannitol 20%	38.1 ± 78.4	41.2 ± 66.2
10-min Control	8.1 ± 30.2	21.9 ± 28.1
20-min Control	4.3 ± 40.1	47.3 ± 65.4

either stimulates or suppresses contractions. The percentage increase in flow rate, bolus volume and peristaltic rate for each increment of diuretic stimulus has also been determined in the mechanically obstructed system.

Table 2.1 shows the comparative values obtained for control and obstructed systems. In the obstructed upper urinary tract the range of bolus volume decreased. Considering the decrease in urine output in this system, the increase in ureteral peristalsis is unlikely to be related to changes in bolus volume. The characteristic changes produced by obstruction are best illustrated in the light of the control measurements. The effects of diuretic stimuli on the obstructed renal pelvis and ureter are illustrated in Fig. 2.11. During the initial 10-min control period, urine flow rate is approximately 0.1 ml/min and the interperistaltic interval approximately 60 s. Following infusion of 5 ml 20% mannitol, flow rate increased to 0.4 ml/min and the bolus volume and the ureteral peristaltic rate doubled in value. When 50 ml 20% mannitol was infused, the initial response was an increase in bolus volume accompanied by a reduction in the ureteral peristaltic rate. However, peristaltic rate changed to bursts of activity with low and high duration of time between peristaltic contractions at flow rates higher than 0.9 ml/min. Interperistaltic intervals ranged from 6 to 70 s and were accompanied by bolus volumes of 0.2–3.0 ml respectively. Interperistaltic intervals of low duration were phasic in occurrence, separated by intervals of approximately 7 s. The distribution of interperistaltic intervals during a

EFFECT OF DIURESIS ON PERISTALSIS AND
BOLUS VOLUME ON HYDRONEPHROTIC KIDNEY

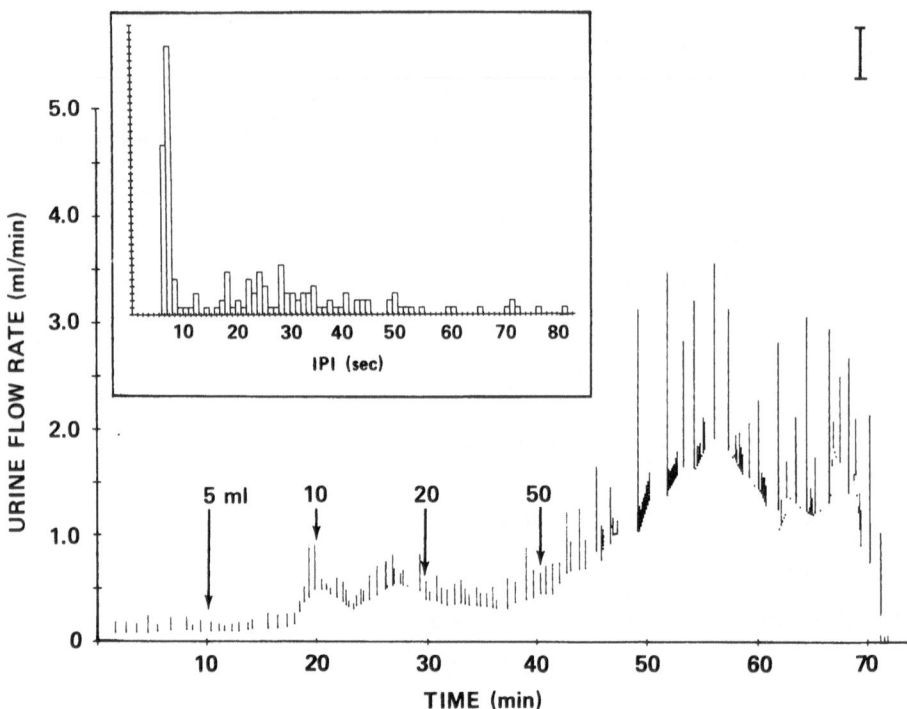

Fig. 2.11. Temporal representation of the relationship between urine flow rate, peristaltic rate and bolus volume. Diuretic stimuli (mannitol 20%) are given as indicated by the *arrows* at 10-min intervals. The amount of mannitol given on each occasion is also shown. The *vertical lines* represent bolus volume; calibration is shown on the right for 1.0 ml. The *spacing* between *vertical lines* represents the interperistaltic interval. This figure demonstrates the accommodation of bolus volume to overall diuresis and illustrates the disruption of regularity in peristalsis. Such disruption is shown as frequent periods of ureteral quiescence followed by large bolus volumes. In addition, the burstlike characteristics of peristalsis in the obstructed system are illustrated. During such activity, high rates of peristalsis occur (IPI ~ 7 s). The histogram shown in the *inset* demonstrates with greater resolution the high rate of ureteral peristalsis caused by diuresis.

17-min continuous recording period is illustrated by the insert histogram in Fig. 2.11. Comparison between the response of the control (Fig. 2.7) and the chronically obstructed upper urinary tract (Fig. 2.11) illustrates the effect of obstruction on both the rhythmicity of peristalsis and the size of bolus volume. The obstructed kidney has an increased range of ureteral peristaltic rate. This increase in range is manifested by higher frequency of ureteric contraction in addition to periods of aperistalsis. As a result of the high peristaltic frequencies encountered, bolus volumes may be very small. Similarly, following a period of aperistalsis bolus volume is large due to the accumulation of urine in the renal pelvis. Neither of these two extremes can be observed in the unobstructed upper urinary tract.

In order to localise the range of the disruptive effects in the obstructed system, it is appropriate to consider some of the properties of peristalsis as recorded

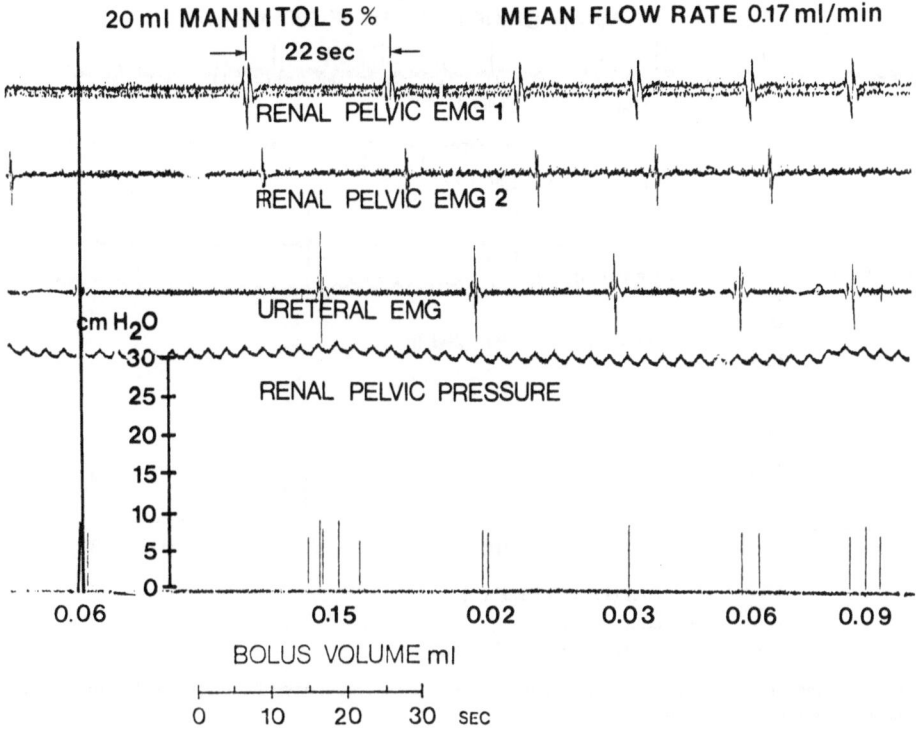

Fig. 2.12. Recording illustrating the transmission characteristics from the renal pelvis to the ureter. The associated bolus volume is indicated, together with renal pelvic pressure. The mean urine flow rate during this period was 0.17 ml/min.

experimentally. Additional information has been obtained by implanting electrodes in the proximal and middle portions of the pelvis, identifying the intrapelvic variation in electrical activity and comparing this with ureteral electrical activity and bolus volume. With these considerations in mind, it is apparent that unlike the control renal pelvis, contraction in the obstructed system is incomplete. The relationship between renal pelvic activity and propagated ureteric contractions is illustrated in Figs. 2.12–2.14. At urine flow rates of 0.2–0.5 ml/min, contractions in the proximal parts of the renal pelvis are invariably propagated into the ureter. Figure 2.12 shows the conduction characteristics of the 'mildly' obstructed preparation at a urine flow rate of 0.17 ml/min. At this flow rate, renal pelvic contractions regularly occur at the rate of 3.0/min and each is associated with a urine bolus. Increase in urine flow rate causes a marked change in the transmission characteristics of renal pelvic contractions by selective blocking of electrical activity.

Figure 2.13 illustrates the electrical transmission of renal pelvic contractions at the urine flow rate of 0.47 ml/min. The rate of proximal pelvic activity has increased from 2/min to over 7/min although not all electrical events are propagated to the electrodes placed in the distal part of the pelvis. Thus, in this particular example, of the 17 contractions detected by the proximal electrodes, only five are propagated distally. In this context, the propagated ureteric contractions are in phase with those occurring in the distal part of the renal pelvis. Further increase in flow rate fails to increase the rate of contraction in the proximal part of the pelvis; the increase in

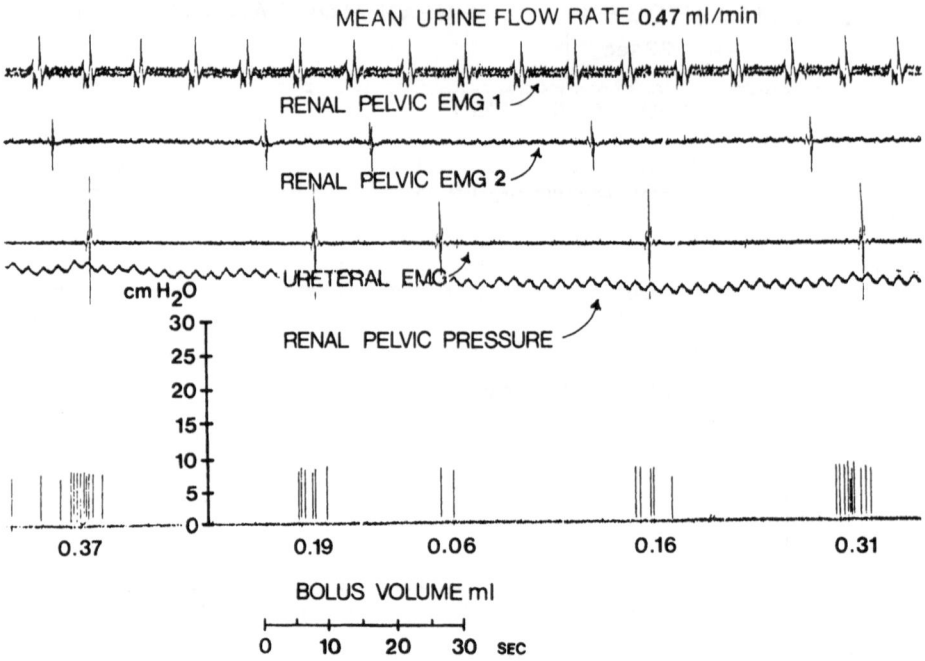

Fig. 2.13. Alteration in the transmission properties and basic frequency of the renal pelvis due to an increase in flow rate to 0.47 ml/min.

fluid flow is accommodated by an increase in bolus volume. In Fig. 2.14 an increase in urine flow rate (0.79 ml/min) causes an additional rise in the frequency of the proximal part of the renal pelvis, which in turn facilitates electrical conduction across the renal pelvis.

In these experiments, the renal pelvic pressure is unaffected by the electrical events occurring in the renal pelvic wall, suggesting that renal pelvic smooth muscle is unable to generate hydrostatic pressures. Figure 2.15 illustrates the result of producing an acute obstruction in the same preparation. Twenty seconds after acute obstruction, the hydrostatic pressure of the pelvis has increased. This overall increase in pressure is oscillatory in nature and is partly associated with electrical activity of the lower region of the pelvis. The peak-to-peak amplitude of the renal pelvic contractions is in the order of 10 cmH$_2$O and is superimposed upon an overall increase in the level of resting pressure. Figure 2.15 also illustrates that in the acutely obstructed renal pelvis, electrical activity from the proximal regions is seemingly better conducted distally. The possibility therefore exists that the distension caused by acute obstruction enhances the conduction properties of the wall of the renal pelvis. In the absence of a propagated bolus (Fig. 2.15), the amplitude from the conducted signal is decreased. In the same experimental preparation, the effect of removing the acute obstruction is illustrated in Fig. 2.16. The pressure in the renal pelvis falls from 60 cmH$_2$O to the value prior to acute obstruction. This pressure reduction is associated with a bolus of 1.33 ml contained by the pelvis during the period of acute obstruction. However, release of the acute obstruction is associated with the return of partial electrical discontinuity between the proximal and distal parts of the pelvis.

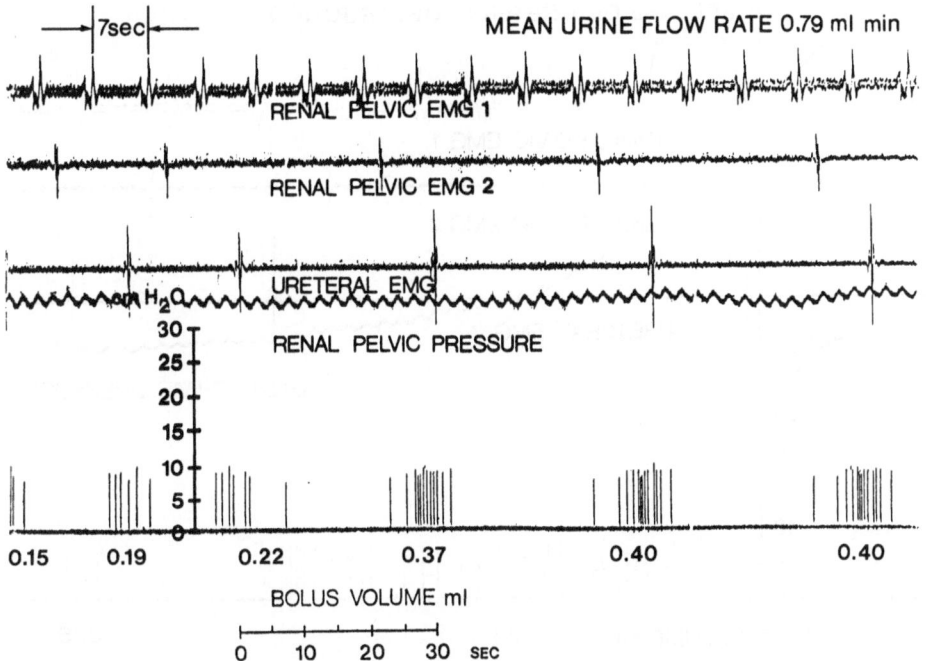

Fig. 2.14. Increase in proximal renal pelvic activity due to higher urine flow rate. Transmission of elevated renal pelvic frequency towards the mid-pelvis and ureter is incomplete.

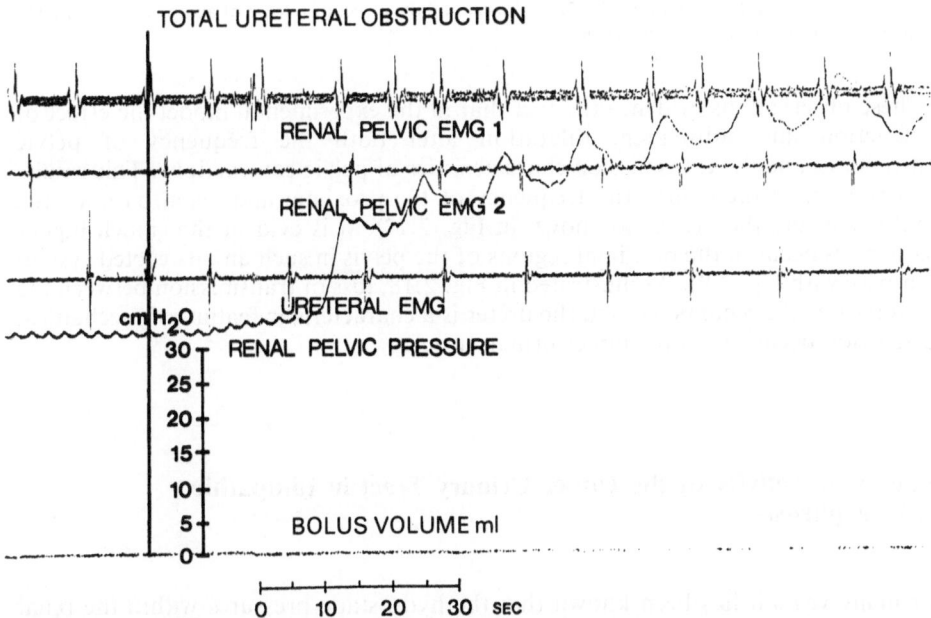

Fig. 2.15. Recording illustrating the effect of acute ureteral obstruction on the proximal and mid-renal pelvis and on the ureter. The onset of obstruction is indicated by the *vertical continuous line*. Note that pelvic contractions are in phase with the electrical activity of the pelvic EMGs and not with those from the proximal region.

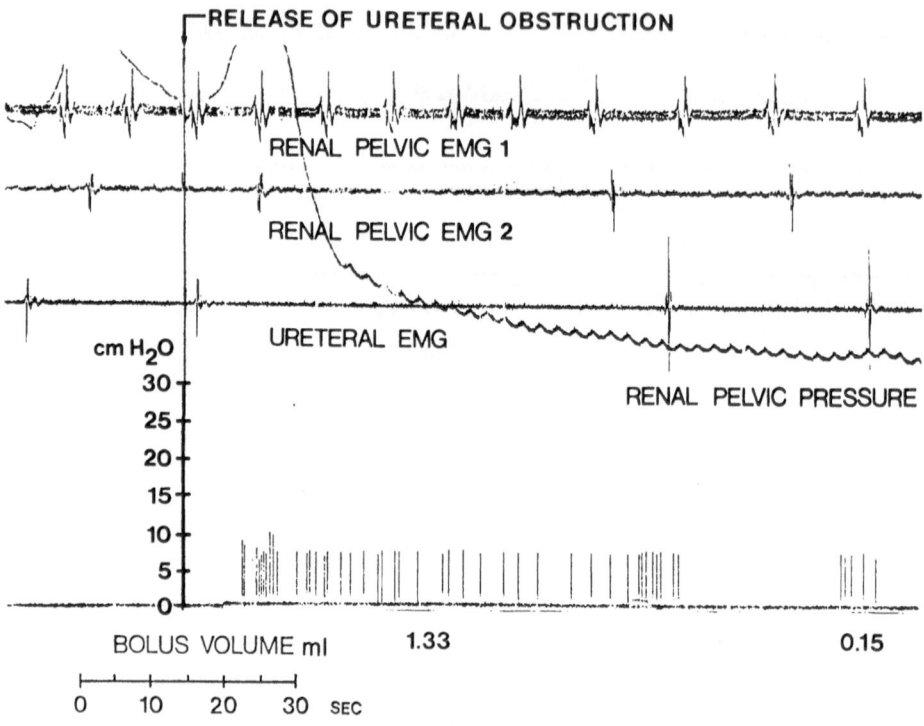

Fig. 2.16. Continuation of data of Fig. 2.15, illustrating the effect of release of acute obstruction. The point of release is indicated by the *arrow*.

These observations evidence the fact that in the experimental model the effect of obstruction and subsequent dilatation alter both the frequency of pelvic contractions and the transmission characteristics of pelvic contractions. This results in disruption of the contractile frequency of the proximal and distal parts of the renal pelvis and the ureter (as shown in Fig. 2.17). It is evident that much higher frequencies occur in the proximal regions of the pelvis in such an obstructed system (compare with Fig. 2.9). As illustrated in Fig. 2.18, loss of transmission between the distal part of the renal pelvis and the ureter is a characteristic feature of mechanical obstruction occurring in the upper urinary tract.

Functional Activity of the Upper Urinary Tract in Idiopathic Hydronephrosis

For many years it has been known that the hydrostatic pressures within the renal pelvis in cases of idiopathic hydronephrosis are in general indistinguishable from those recorded in the normal system (Underwood 1937; Kiil 1957; Djurhuus et al. 1976b, c). In the experimental model, it has also been established that pressures in the renal pelvis following long-term mechanical obstruction of the ureter are not

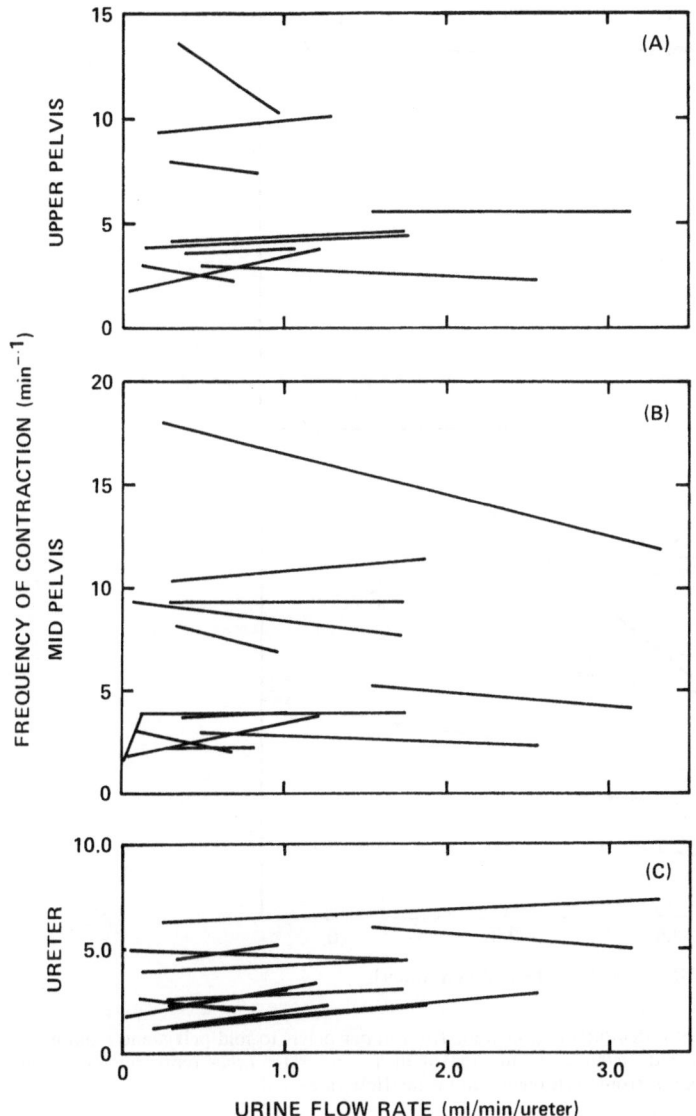

Fig. 2.17. Regional variation of the frequency of contraction of the obstructed system with respect to urine flow rate. *Lines* represent regression equations over the range of measured urine flow rate and rate of peristalsis.

significantly different from those obtained in the normal (Schweitzer 1973; Djurhuus et al. 1976a). Thus, measurement of renal pelvic pressures alone in clinical hydronephrosis plays a relatively minor role in the evaluation of this condition.

During the past 10 years, a variety of new methods has been introduced in efforts to provide data which are of value in the clinical evaluation of upper urinary tract obstruction. Such methods include dynamic pressure measurements obtained percutaneously or intraoperatively from the renal pelvis during constant perfusion

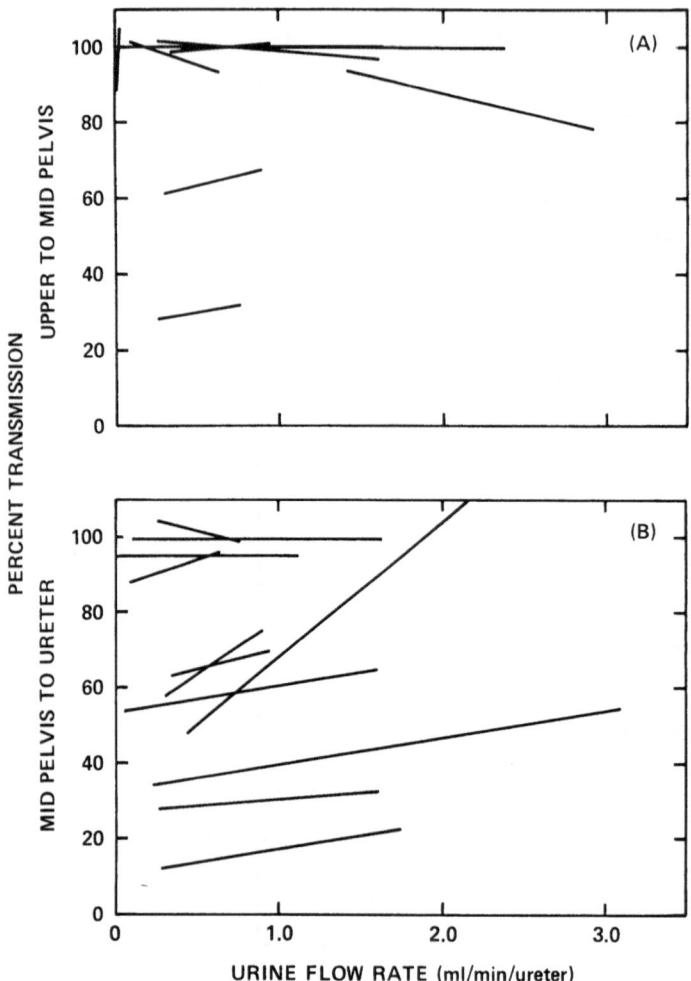

Fig. 2.18. Transmission of electrical action potentials from upper pelvis to mid-pelvis and from mid-pelvis to ureter in the obstructed system as a function of urine flow rate. *Lines* represent regression equations of percent transmission from each region and urine flow rate.

(see Chaps. 5 and 6). A perfusion rate of 5–10 ml/min has been recommended while the pressures in the renal pelvis are being recorded. The test divides idiopathic hydronephrosis into two clearly separate groups: one associated with a pronounced pressure increase while, in the second, the pressure remains low (Fig. 2.19). The clinical significance of this differentiation remains uncertain since long-term follow-up studies have not yet been reported.

Other new methods of assessing obstruction in the upper urinary tract include the estimation of changes in the area of the renal pelvis during intravenous pyelography (Whitfield et al. 1979), and the use of isotope renography (see Chap. 4), both procedures involving the administration of diuretics. An increase in pelvic area of less than 22% or a rapid decline on the excretion curve in diuresis renography are believed to indicate a non-obstructed system. While both methods have the

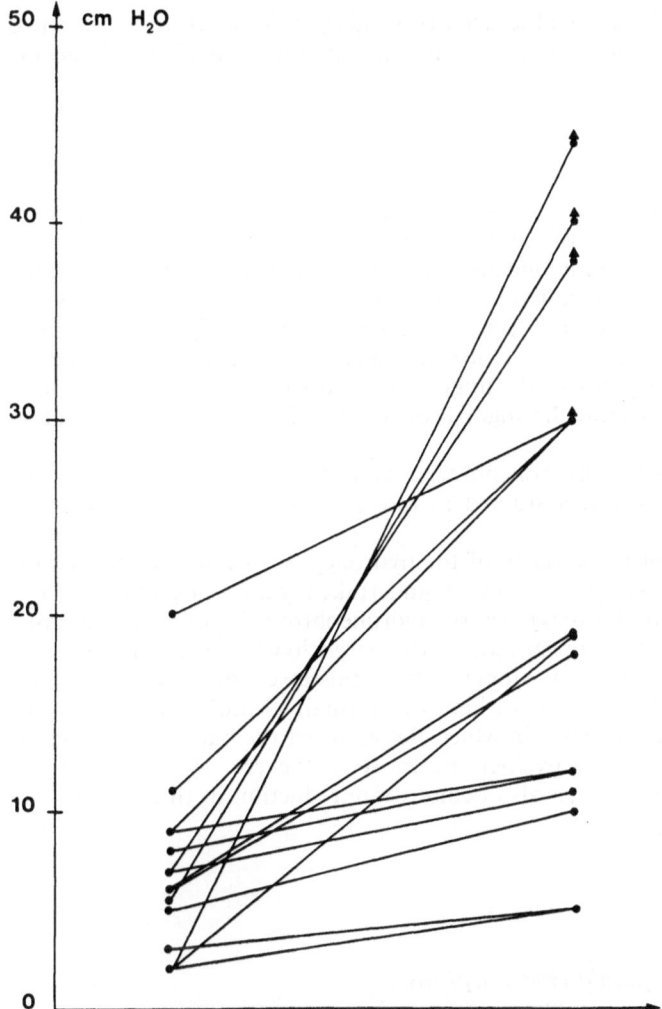

Fig. 2.19. Constant perfusion provocation in 15 cases of idiopathic hydronephrosis. Infusion rate, 8 cm³/min. Six patients showed a continuous increase in pressure during the investigation. The remainder stabilised at pressures below 20 cmH₂O.

advantage of being relatively non-invasive, the results are dependent upon the capability of the kidney in question to produce urine. Therefore, the outcome of these tests must be equivocal in cases in which the function of the kidney is severely impaired.

These methods are designed basically to be of value in the clinical management of idiopathic hydronephrosis and do not provide information on the pathogenesis of the disease. Investigations of the aetiological factors of the disease must focus on urine transport in the system and thereby on the peristaltic activity of the upper urinary tract.

Recently, a method for simultaneously recording pressure waves in the renal pelvis together with measurement of electrical activity from the pelvis and ureter has been designed to study the peristaltic activity in idiopathic hydronephrosis. The method and the results obtained with this technique will now be considered in detail.

Method

Platinum recording electrodes are sutured at selected sites to the wall of the renal pelvis and ureter at the time of surgical exposure of the obstructed system. Intrapelvic pressure is measured by means of a fluid-filled catheter introduced into the renal pelvis either by direct puncture or by insertion through the parenchyma. Pressure values and electromyographic activity are recorded during restricted fluid administration (1 ml saline.$kg^{-1}.h^{-1}$). Once baseline data have been obtained under standard conditions, the response of the upper urinary tract to either an intravenous injection of a diuretic (frusemide 0.5 mg/kg) or to a renal pelvic infusion of saline (8 ml/min) is determined.

All degrees of idiopathic hydronephrosis have been investigated. Normal contralateral upper urinary tracts studied at the time of surgery have served as controls.

In the following account the severity of the hydronephrosis has been judged on the basis of intravenous urography (IVU) undertaken with Urografin (76% 1 ml/kg). With this method the diagnosis of hydronephrosis is restricted to cases which show alterations in the appearance of the parenchyma. Therefore, a large-volume pelvis (pelviectasia) in a kidney which possesses papillae of normal appearance is considered to be a variant of normal. 'Mild' and 'moderate' hydronephrosis refers to those cases in which flattening of the papillae, or absence of papillary protrusions into the pyelogram, are seen. 'Severe' hydronephrosis is used to describe those cases which also demonstrate reduction in thickness of the parenchyma.

Results

Peristaltic Activity in Idiopathic Hydronephrosis

On the basis of this classification, control renal pelves (including pelviectasia) show a pattern of peristaltic activity similar to that registered in the normal pig. Electromyographic activity recorded from electrodes placed adjacent to the renal hilum crosses the renal pelvis and is detected in the pelviureteric region. The transmission of this activity occurs with a constant time lag between the proximal and distal leads. Each electromyographic event is accompanied by a pressure wave of uniform shape, the maximal amplitude of which corresponds to the arrival of electromyographic activity at electrodes situated in the pelviureteric region. The activity registered in the pelviureteric region is usually transmitted to the ureter. Electromyographic activity arising spontaneously within the ureter is not observed in control material (Fig. 2.20).

Mild and Moderate Hydronephrosis

Registration of renal pelvic electromyographic activity in these cases shows evidence of discoordination between the proximal and distal pelvic electrodes. Activity

NORMAL PERISTALSIS

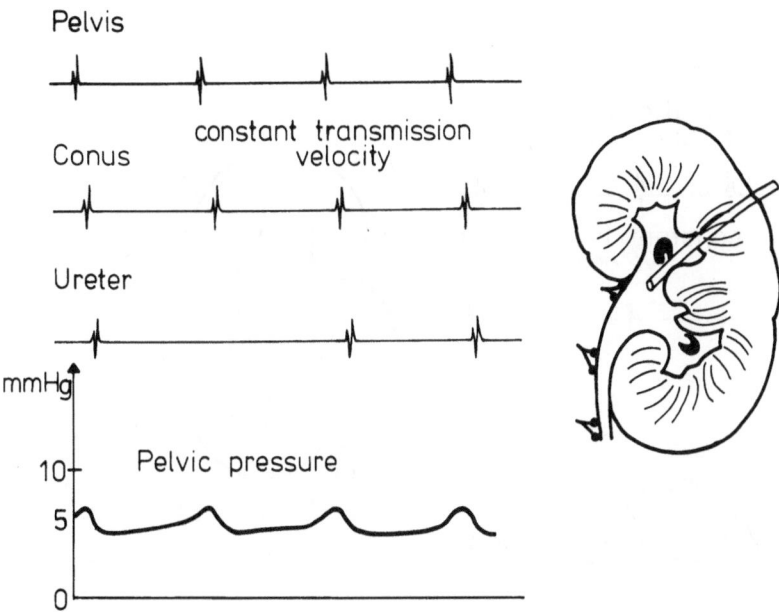

Pelvis

Conus

constant transmission
velocity

Ureter

mmHg

10

Pelvic pressure

5

0

Fig. 2.20. Schematic drawing of the method of investigation together with findings in the normal human pelvis and ureter. Bipolar surface electrodes are sutured to selected regions of the renal pelvis and to the ureter below the pelviureteric region. Activity recorded from the proximal electrodes is transmitted to the pelviureteric region at constant transmission velocity. The pressure waves measured in the renal pelvis during stable conditions are of uniform shape. At low urine flow, increase in baseline pressure is observed only during renal pelvic contractions. At high urine flow, the pressure increase occurs before the onset of a contraction. Note that the EMG activity recorded from the electrode in the pelviureteric region coincides with the maximum value of the pressure trace.

recorded proximally may precede, coincide with or follow electrical events measured by the distal electrodes. Consistent with this finding, the renal pelvic pressure waves are not uniform in shape and variations in duration and amplitude occur. However, the transmission of peristaltic activity from the pelviureteric region into the ureter is similar to that observed in normal upper urinary tracts. Thus, the alterations in peristaltic activity in case of mild and moderate idiopathic hydronephrosis are similar to the events which have been induced experimentally following long-term partial ureteric obstruction (Fig. 2.21).

Severe Idiopathic Hydronephrosis

In these patients, peristaltic activity measured electrically is continuously uncoordinated between the renal pelvic and the ureteric electrodes (Fig. 2.22). Consistent with these findings, pressure waves are usually not detected in the renal pelvis.

MILDLY ABNORMAL
PERISTALSIS

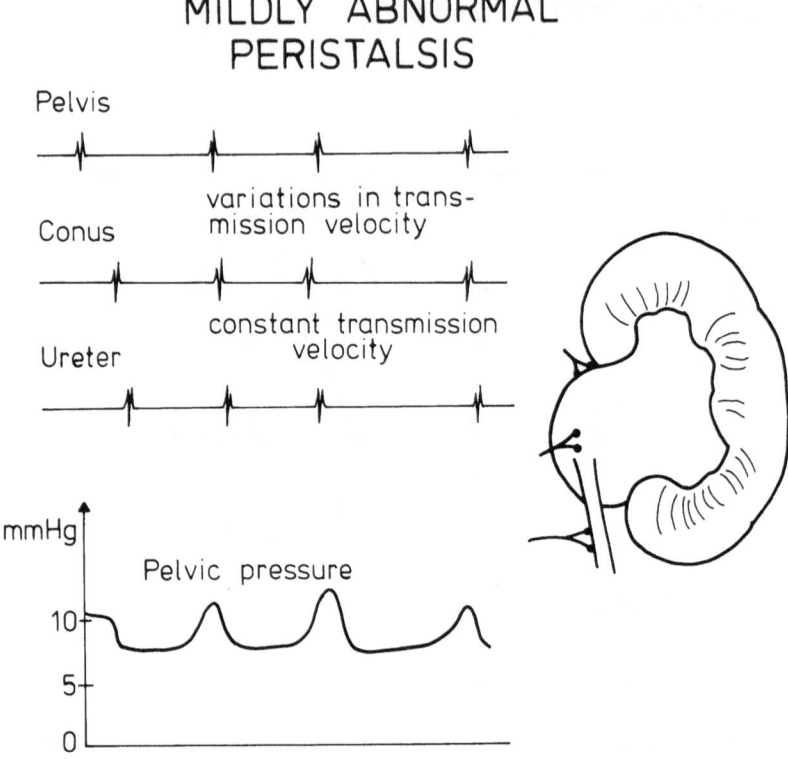

Pelvis

variations in trans-
mission velocity

Conus

constant transmission
velocity

Ureter

mmHg

Pelvic pressure

10

5

0

Fig. 2.21. Observations recorded in a mild case of hydronephrosis. Activity recorded proximally precedes, coincides with, or follows EMG activity registered by the distal electrode. The activity of the pelviureteric region is transmitted to the ureter as in the normal system, however. Note that the pressure waves recorded from the renal pelvis vary in amplitude and duration.

Discussion

From the foregoing, it is evident that in mild and moderate idiopathic hydronephrosis disruption of electrical transmission occurs between the proximal and distal parts of the renal pelvis. In such cases however, coordination between the pelviureteric region and the ureter is maintained. These findings are consistent with the morphological alterations which occur in the pelvic wall in idiopathic hydronephrosis, and which do not extend into the adjacent, apparently normal segment of ureter (Chap. 1). It is only in the severe cases that the disease seems to alter the functional coordination between the pelvis and the ureter.

The similarity between the results obtained from experimental long-term ureteric obstruction and from idiopathic hydronephrosis suggest that an obstruction to urine flow (possibly in the pelviureteric region) occurs in the latter condition. The aetiology of this obstruction remains unknown. Possible contenders include a subtle organic or mechanical obstruction, or an abnormal muscle arrangement which alters the cable properties of ureteric smooth muscle bundles.

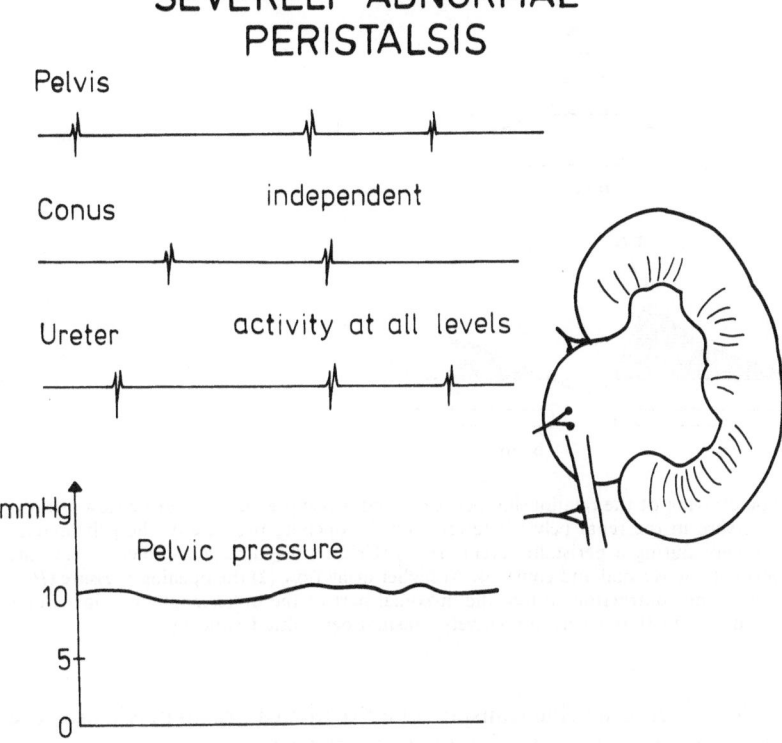

Fig. 2.22. Observations recorded in a patient with severe hydronephrosis. Total uncoordination of peristaltic activity is observed between all the recording electrodes. The pressure waves are of low amplitude and difficult to distinguish from baseline pressure.

Urine transport from the renal pelvis to the ureter necessitates that the pelviureteric region opens to receive a urine bolus. Opening of the pelviureteric region is probably related to the pressure value within the renal pelvis. In studies of low urine flow, opening of the pelviureteric region is accomplished only during peristaltic activity. At higher urine output, filling of the proximal ureter also occurs prior to contraction of the renal pelvis (Fig. 2.23). That a resistance to flow occurs in the pelviureteric region has been shown in studies in which urine is intermittently drained (via a catheter) from the normal renal pelvis. Complete drainage of fluid from the renal pelvis results in a small reduction in intrapelvic pressure. When the pressure is raised by reducing the drainage through the intrapelvic catheter, the pelvic pressure increase is sufficient to enable fluid transport into the ureter (Djurhuus 1977).

In idiopathic hydronephrosis it seems likely that the pressure required to open the pelviureteric region is increased. Thus, increased pelvic peristaltic work is required to transport urine and this necessitates an increase in baseline renal pelvic pressure. In this context, when idiopathic hydronephrosis is classified on the basis of IVU (Table 2.2) a slight increase in baseline pressure is noted when normals are compared with mild and moderate cases, and when the latter are compared with severe cases. It

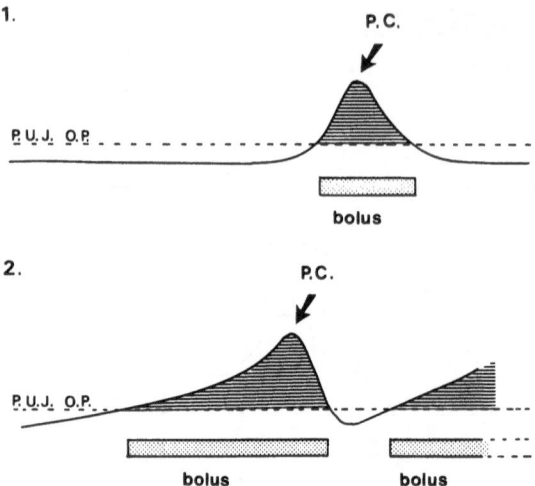

Fig. 2.23. Schematic drawing of the relationship between renal pelvic pressure and urine flow. At low urine flow (**1**) the pressure in the renal pelvis is lower than the opening pressure of the pelviureteral junction (*PUJ OP*) except during a peristaltic event (*P.C.*). Urine transport occurs solely during the contraction: the bolus volume is small and constant. At higher urine flow (**2**) the opening pressure (*PUJ OP*) is exceeded prior to the contraction so that the proximal part of the ureter contains urine. Bolus volume varies with urine production despite a relatively constant peristaltic frequency.

may be that in order to achieve urine transport the rise in mean renal pelvic pressure correlates with the degree of severity of the hydronephrosis.

In states of high urine output, the proximal segment of the normal ureter contains fluid prior to the arrival of a renal pelvic contraction (Djurhuus and Constantinou 1979). The length of this segment of ureter varies according to urine production and is independent of pelvic contraction (the latter occurs at the constant pacing frequency of the renal pelvis). In idiopathic hydronephrosis passive filling of the ureter prior to renal pelvic contraction is hindered. This results in the formation of smaller bolus volumes as urine production varies. In pronounced obstruction, more of the bolus has to be launched during individual pelvic contractions. Therefore, in contrast to the normal system, increased urine transport in idiopathic hydronephrosis is accomplished by an increase in the mean peristaltic frequency.

Bolus volumes measured during moderate urine flow rates in idiopathic hydronephrosis have not yet been determined. Determination of this parameter remains as a difficult technical problem although the preliminary use of less invasive methods has shown promise for the future (Djurhuus and Constantinou 1979).

In the transitional phase culminating in maximal urine flow rates renal pelvic contractions occur at frequencies similar to those of the calyces. Under these conditions the renal pelvis frequently launches boli of small uniform size. This high-frequency activity associated with small stroke volumes is an expedient method in the transportation of urine. In the normal system, this state occurs only during rapid variations in fluid flow. As soon as the stimulus decreases, the peristaltic rate falls to that of the pelvic pacemaker— the increased urine production is then achieved by enlargement of bolus volume.

The response can be observed experimentally in long-term ureteric obstruction even during constant rates of urine production. In clinical hydronephrosis this effect

Table 2.2. Intrapelvic baseline pressure in idiopathic hydronephrosis

		Intrapelvic pressures
Patients above the age of 15		
Normal (or pelviectasia)		
	Total 8	5.7 ± 1.6 mmHg
Mild and moderate		
	Total 28	7.0 ± 3.6 mmHg
Severe		
	Total 11	9.1 ± 3.8 mmHg
Patients below the age of 15		
Mild and moderate		
	Total 5	5.4 ± 4.6 mmHg
Severe		
	Total 7	10.7 ± 5.8 mmHg

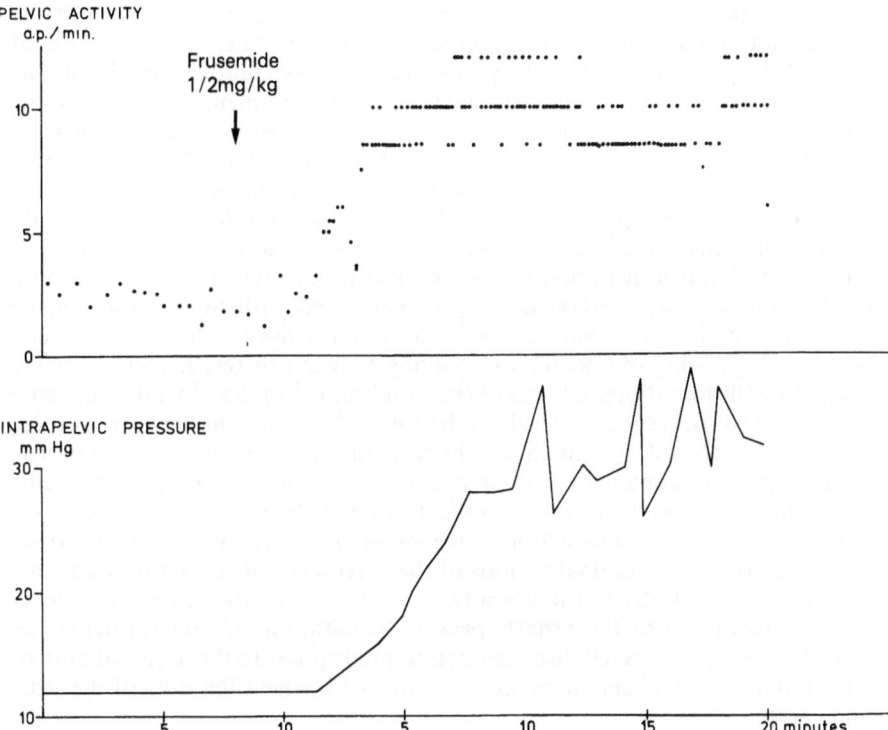

Fig. 2.24. Investigation of renal pelvic peristaltic activity and intrapelvic pressure in a patient with hydronephrosis. The frequency of peristaltic activity is 2–4/min prior to the induction of diuresis. During diuresis the pelvic pressure rises and the frequency of peristaltic activity is increased to 10–12/min. This frequency is maximal and similar in value to that of the renal calyces. This maximum frequency is sustained throughout the period of the renal pelvic pressure rise.

is observed (Fig. 2.24) when the system is provoked either by a high diuretic load or by constant fluid perfusion. In these conditions coupling of peristaltic activity between the different parts of the renal pelvis and ureter is often observed. However, such high peristaltic frequencies are relatively inefficient at achieving adequate urine transport.

Urine output at the high rates used in perfusion studies is seldom achieved in the normal daily life of the patient with hydronephrosis. At these lower urine flow rates the pressure needed to open the system becomes the factor of paramount importance. The present investigation has revealed a difference (albeit small) in the renal pelvic baseline pressure in different groups of hydronephrotic patients. This pressure differential may prove to be the most important parameter in future investigations on the dynamics of the upper urinary tract in idiopathic hydronephrosis.

Summary of the Physiology of the Hydronephrotic Upper Urinary Tract

Chronic obstruction of the upper urinary tract disrupts the mechanism of coordination between the proximal and distal parts of the renal pelvis. The outcome results in the dissociation of the proximal regions of the pelvis from those of the distal pelvis and the ureter. During increases in urine flow rate, the rate of contraction of the proximal part of the pelvis increases. By contrast, the distal part of the pelvis maintains a level of activity which is of lower frequency than that of the proximal regions. Since ureteral peristalsis and the associated bolus are in phase at the same frequency as the electrical activity of the distal pelvis, the latter can be considered as the region which paces ureteric activity. Thus, the net effect of chronic obstruction results in the apparent loss of conduction through the renal pelvic wall.

These controlled investigations show that obstruction and hydronephrosis alter the regulating mechanism of initiation and conduction of ureteral peristalsis. With moderate hydronephrosis, ureteral activity is associated with bursts followed by long periods of aperistalsis. Diuresis tends to establish normal levels of ureteric rhythmicity by improving the degree of coupling between different regions of the renal pelvis. In addition, diuretic loads over 3–5 ml.min^{-1} ureter^{-1} tend to increase the rate of peristalsis to frequency levels in the calyceal system. On the basis of these observations, the calyceal system in the hydronephrotic system can temporarily become the triggering mechanism of ureteral peristalsis. Finally, the electrical events within the renal pelvis and the ureter indicate that in hydronephrosis there is a failure of transmission of contractions throughout the renal pelvis. Thus, renal pelvic contractions in the proximal regions of the pelvis are only partially conducted to the ureter. As a result discoordination between regions of the renal pelvis occur leading to the disruption of the orderly process of initiation of ureteral peristalsis from the proximal regions. Such discoordination predisposes to the accumulation of urine in the renal pelvis and enhances the possibility of further dilatation of the renal pelvis and calyces.

References

Constantinou CE (1974) Renal pelvic pacemaker control of ureteral peristaltic rate. Am J Physiol 226: 1413–1416

Constantinou CE, Neubarth J, Mensah-Dwuman M (1978) Frequency gradient in the autorhythmicity of the pyeloureteral pacemaker system. Experientia 34: 614–615

Djurhuus JC (1977) Dynamics of upper urinary tract III. The activity of renal pelvis during pressure variations. Invest Urol 14: 475

Djurhuus JC, Constantinou CE (1979) Assessment of pyeloureteral function using a flow velocity and cross-sectional diameter probe. Invest Urol 17: 103–107

Djurhuus JC, Nerstrom B, Gyrd-Hansen N, Rask-Andersen H (1976a) Experimental hydronephrosis. An electrophysiologic investigation before and after release of obstruction. Acta Chir Scand (Suppl) 472: 17

Djurhuus JC, Nerstrom B, Iversen-Hansen R, Rask-Andersen H (1976b) Incomplete ureteral duplication. Electromyographic and manometric investigation. Scand J Urol Nephrol 10: 111

Djurhuus JC, Berstrom B, Rask-Andersen H (1976c) Dynamics of upper urinary tract in man. Preoperative electrophysiological findings in patients with manifest or suspected hydronephrosis. Acta Chir Scand (Suppl) 472: 49

Gosling JA, Constantinou CE (1976) The origin and propagation of upper urinary tract contraction waves — a new in vitro methodology. Experientia 32: 666–667

Hannappel J, Lutzeyer W (1978) Pacemaker localization in the renal pelvis of the unicalyceal kidney. In vitro study in the rabbit. Eur Urol 4: 192–194

Kiil F (1957) The function of the ureter and renal pelvis. University Press, Oslo

Schweitzer FAW (1973) Intra-pelvic pressure and renal function studies in experimental chronic partial ureteric obstruction. Br J Urol 45: 2

Underwood WE (1937) Recent observations on the pathology of hydronephrosis. Proc R Soc Med 30: 817

Weiss RM (1976) Initiation and organization of ureteral peristalsis. Urol Surv 26: 2–17

Weiss RM (1979) Clinical implications of ureteral physiology. J Urol 121: 401–413

Whitfield HN, Britton KE, Hendry WF, Wickham JEA (1979) Frusemide intravenous urography in the diagnosis of pelviureteric junction obstruction. Br J Urol 51: 445–448

3. The Intravenous Urogram in Idiopathic Hydronephrosis

T. Sherwood

This chapter outlines the place of conventional radiology in the diagnosis and management of idiopathic hydronephrosis. The shortcomings of the intravenous urogram (IVU) have given rise to radionuclide and pressure studies, but the IVU, nevertheless, remains the common initial study which may raise the question of hydronephrosis in any patient (Fig. 3.1).

Gross hydronephrosis with severe renal atrophy and functional impairment is the only part of the problem where ultrasound has an important diagnostic role. In the child or adult with a poorly excreting kidney of normal size, ultrasound is the obvious next investigation. If the functional impairment is the result of obstruction, ultrasound will demonstrate the dilated pelvicalyceal system. A plain film of the abdomen is still needed however— if a large staghorn calculus plugging distended calyces is responsible, ultrasound may be misleading.

For the more common problem of patients suspected of having hydronephrosis because of unilateral loin pain, the mere demonstration of pelvicalyceal dilatation is not enough. The central question is: does the renal abnormality account for the patient's symptoms, and therefore demand surgery? The IVU is able to distinguish between other causes of unilateral loin pain, and to give some information about urine transport. For these reasons it is likely to remain the first radiological investigation for these patients.

Acute and Chronic Obstruction

The IVU is very useful in the diagnosis of acute obstruction. The radiological signs of this state are known well enough: increasingly dense nephrogram and delayed, distended pyelogram (Fig. 3.2). A normal IVU excludes acute urinary tract obstruction.

The IVU is of limited value in the diagnosis of chronic obstruction because the functional derangements are different (Sherwood 1980). If a dilated upper urinary tract is found, is this a sign of an unimportant structural aberration, or of correctable obstruction? The diagnostic problem of the chronically dilated upper urinary tract is made worse by the intermittent acute obstructive character of idiopathic hydronephrosis. Some of the IVU modifications described at the end of this chapter exploit these facts by determining whether acute obstruction can be induced. The use of such methods may transfer the questions to an area where the IVU can give confident answers.

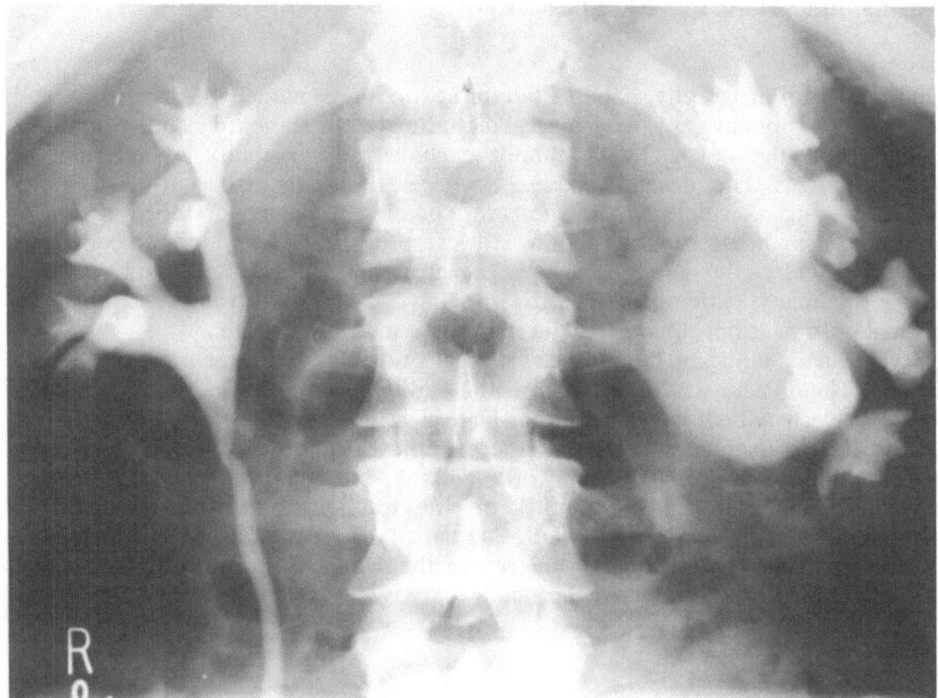

Fig. 3.1. A dilated left pelvicalyceal system, suggestive of idiopathic hydronephrosis. Question: obstruction or non-obstructed dilatation?

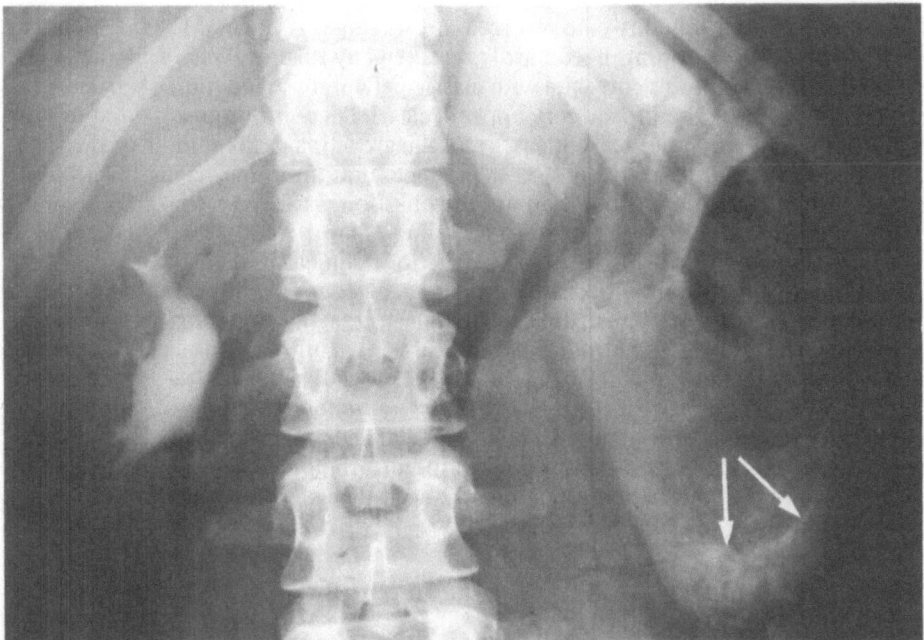

Fig. 3.2. Acute on chronic obstruction. Dense left nephrogram with 'calyceal crescents' (*arrows*) at the rim of dilated non-opacified calyces.

Normal and Abnormal Standard IVUs

On the basis of urography, patients fall into two groups, namely those who do, and those who do not have any pelvicalyceal dilatation on the standard examination. It is evident that the normal IVU cannot exclude the possibility of intermittent hydronephrosis. The ideal IVU series showing a funnel-shaped renal pelvis/upper ureter working as a single dynamic unit, with no discernible pelviureteric junction, is an unlikely candidate for obstruction. However, there is now widespread consensus that no pelviureteric junction can ever be pronounced to be immutably perfect. There are many patients on record who have progressed from such apparent normality to develop obvious pelviureteric junction obstruction.

Even when a modestly dilated pelvicalyceal system is found, the issue is far from certain. The difficulty is accentuated if the oddity is a chance finding in a middle-aged or elderly patient whose nephrons have clearly survived for many years in this setting of 'hydronephrosis'. Time-honoured radiological observations such as rapid ureteric filling are probably still worth making, but it must be recognised that assessment of urine transport relies on the fraction-of-a-second observations documented during the IVU. A whole standard IVU series adds up to a second or two of a patient's horizontal life: the rest of the urinary 24 h (most of them spent upright) should not be inferred too readily.

Clinical Judgement and the Standard IVU

A few problems can obviously be resolved at this stage. A normal IVU in a patient with unconvincing symptoms need hardly be taken any further. Where characteristic severe unilateral symptoms correlate with classic pelviureteric junction obstruction as seen on the IVU, the road to surgery appears clear. There is disagreement about the proportions between these clearcut cases and the grey area in the middle of the field. Even in the necessarily special referral practice at Cambridge, clear black/white cases are found. But more often than not the question is raised: is this an obstructed kidney or is it not?

In most cases of suspected chronic obstruction, clinical judgement and the IVU are not enough. The standard examination can of course be modified in order to look further into the special problems of intermittent hydronephrosis. These are documented below, but it should be emphasised that they are not necessarily the most appropriate next diagnostic step. If the patient is seen after an equivocal standard IVU has already been performed, a radionuclide study at this stage is generally required. The diuresis IVU is best carried out as part of the original examination; this implies close radiological monitoring of all IVUs in progress (the tailored urogram). The patient should only need a second 'special' IVU if doubt remains after these initial steps.

IVU Modifications

The Standard Follow-up IVU

This is mentioned only to be condemned. 'Let's have another look in 6 months' is still much practised when in doubt. Patients are finally sent on with a letter saying 'although she has had three IVUs, the diagnosis remains in doubt.' The implied faith in repeated offerings to exactly the same uncertain deity is clearly absurd as well as expensive!

The Diuresis IVU

Most sensibly, this forms part II of a standard IVU carried out for suspected hydronephrosis. The patient is given a short-acting intravenous diuretic (e.g., frusemide) after the baseline nephrogram/pyelogram, i.e., 5–10 min after the start. An immediate fast diuresis puts the pelviureteric junction under stress: whether the renal pelvis can cope may be observed fluoroscopically, or recorded on film taken over the next 5–15 min. Considerable distension of the pelvis, with failure to wash out its contrast-laden urine, possibly accompanied by typical loin pain, are of course obvious signs of significant hydronephrosis (Fig. 3.3). Alternatively there may be rapid, bilaterally symmetric wash-out of pelvic contents, indicating a normal urine transport system.

Whitfield et al. (1979) have studied cases in whom less clear-cut results have been obtained. These authors related radionuclide studies and upper urinary tract pressure measurements to the increase in area of the renal pelvis induced during the IVU. They found a 22% renal pelvis area increase to be a useful watershed figure

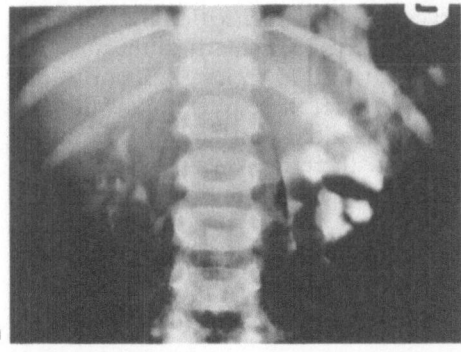
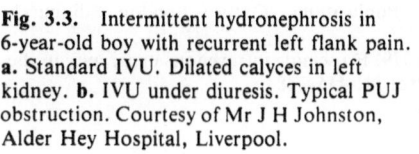
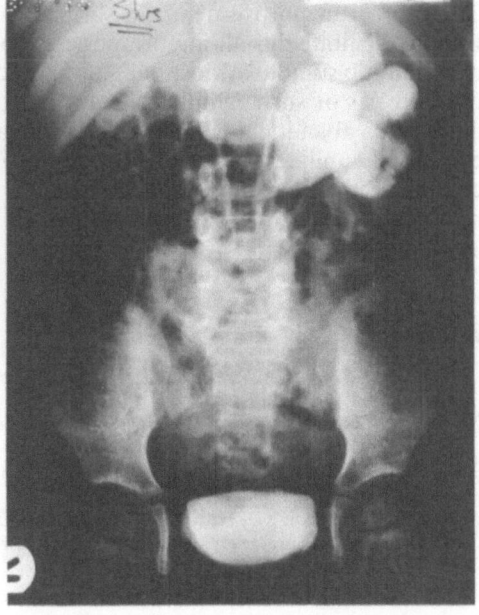

Fig. 3.3. Intermittent hydronephrosis in 6-year-old boy with recurrent left flank pain. **a.** Standard IVU. Dilated calyces in left kidney. **b.** IVU under diuresis. Typical PUJ obstruction. Courtesy of Mr J H Johnston, Alder Hey Hospital, Liverpool.

which aided the distinction between normal and abnormal. Recalculation of their figures in terms of sensitivity and specificity (true-positive and true-negative rates) suggests that the diuresis IVU is a sensitive indicator of obstruction. False-negative rates are therefore low, but some false-positive results will occur.

It is fair to say, therefore, that the diuresis IVU is well worth performing as part of the patient's first IVU, but not as a special examination in the doubtful case. Diuresis radionuclide studies then appear more apt.

The Acute Pain IVU

This is probably the simplest and most reliable approach to the problem. It makes use of the well placed confidence in the IVU as an arbiter of acute obstruction. The patient is instructed to rush himself to the X-ray department for an immediate IVU as soon as an attack of pain begins. An examination carried out under these circumstances has every chance of being decisive. Davies et al. (1978) have shown that this tactic can uncover hydronephroses that have resisted detection by the diuresis IVU. They also stress the importance of upright films.

The only reason that this practice is not widespread is the logistic difficulty of getting the subject onto an X-ray table at 5-10 minutes' notice during his ordinary outpatient life. It is undoubtedly worth attempting in the difficult case.

Conclusions

Most patients with unilateral loin symptoms will be submitted to an IVU. Given close clinico-radiological understanding, this is a useful start to solving the patient's diagnostic problem. Further tests will often be needed to decide whether a doubtful case of hydronephrosis demands surgical intervention. Confidence that the IVU can usually facilitate this all-important decision is misplaced, particularly in the absence of a diuretic stimulus. Most patients should not be denied or enticed into operation on the basis of such fallible evidence. At the same time, these reservations do not allow us to abandon a useful, reasonably safe investigation, which may reveal other causes of unilateral loin pain. The IVU must therefore wear its new hat circumspectly: the dilated upper urinary tract needs a critical but not nihilistic radiological eye.

References

Davies P, Woods KA, Evans CM, Gray WM, Kulatilake AE (1978) The value of provocative and acute urography in patients with intermittent loin pain. Br J Urol 50: 227–232

Sherwood T (1980) Uroradiology. Blackwell Scientific Publications, Oxford London Edinburgh Melbourne, pp 222 and 242

Whitfield HN, Britton KE, Hendry WF, Wickham JEA (1979) Frusemide intravenous urography in the diagnosis of pelviureteric junction obstruction. Br J Urol 51: 445–448

4. Nuclear Medicine

P.H. O'Reilly and E.W. Lupton

The introduction of the ^{131}I-hippuran renogram by Taplin and his colleagues (Taplin et al. 1956) led to an initial surge of interest in the technique amongst urologists and nephrologists. This was short-lived, however, since the initial capabilities of the probe renogram could not match the aspirations and expectations of clinicians. The method remained a useful procedure in renovascular hypertension, and continued to find a place in the evaluation of obstructive uropathy in some centres, but in general there was a certain amount of disillusionment with nuclear medicine in urological investigation until the advent of the gamma camera.

Previous studies of renography in hydronephrosis illustrate this well. In 1969, Davies, Jones and Croft examined 20 patients after pyeloplasty, and concluded that 80% could be said to show improved tubular function (though only 50% showed improved drainage), yet Otnes and his colleagues (1975) demonstrated functional improvement in only eight of 24 patients (33%). Roberts, Slade and Jefferey (1972), examining 75 cases over a 3-year period, were able to show little renogram evidence of change in most cases, yet Tveter et al. (1975) demonstrated post-operative improvement in 75% of 21 patients at 3 months, and almost all at 1 year. More recently, Karlberg (1976) concluded on the basis of 41 examinations that the longer one left the renography post-operatively, the better the functional improvement demonstrable; however, he was unable to comment on any improvement in drainage.

None of these series was concerned with the pre-operative evaluation of the dilated renal pelvis, and all reached different conclusions. The problems involved can be seen in retrospect to have been three-fold. Firstly, the gamma camera was not available so accurate quantitation was difficult; secondly, there was no standardised protocol for the radionuclide evaluations and thirdly, there was need for a clearer understanding of the urodynamic events occurring in the renal pelvis. The only attempt to overcome these deficiencies was that made by Johnston and Kathel (1972) who used the technique of analogue computer simulation to investigate drainage from post-pyeloplasty cases, and demonstrated improvement in 29 of 32 cases, compared with only nine by standard renography.

It was becoming clear during these years that the equation of dilatation of the upper tract with obstruction was simply wrong and it is now accepted that the two are mutually independent. Many examples exist, which are only too familiar to urologists and radiologists, where dilatation occurs in the absence of obstruction, and they need not be enumerated again. However, to make renography meaningful, it is essential to appreciate that *any* situation which results in retention of tracer in the field of a detector will produce a curve indistinguishable from obstruction. The stasis occurring in the isotope mixing chamber of a dilated renal pelvis is a particularly good example and accounts for many of the technical frustrations experienced by early investigators (Fig. 4.1).

It is against this background that two new radionuclide techniques using the gamma camera have emerged for the assessment of such patients— parenchymal transit time studies and diuresis renography.

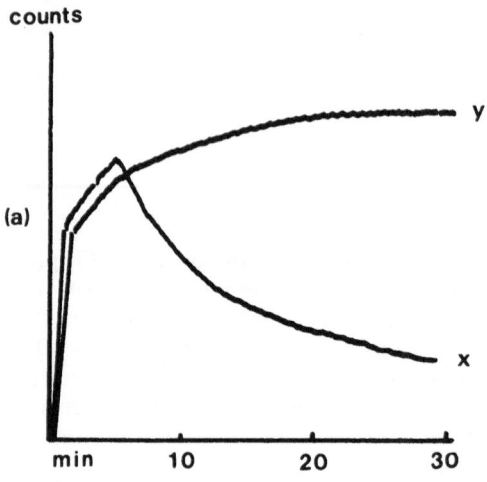

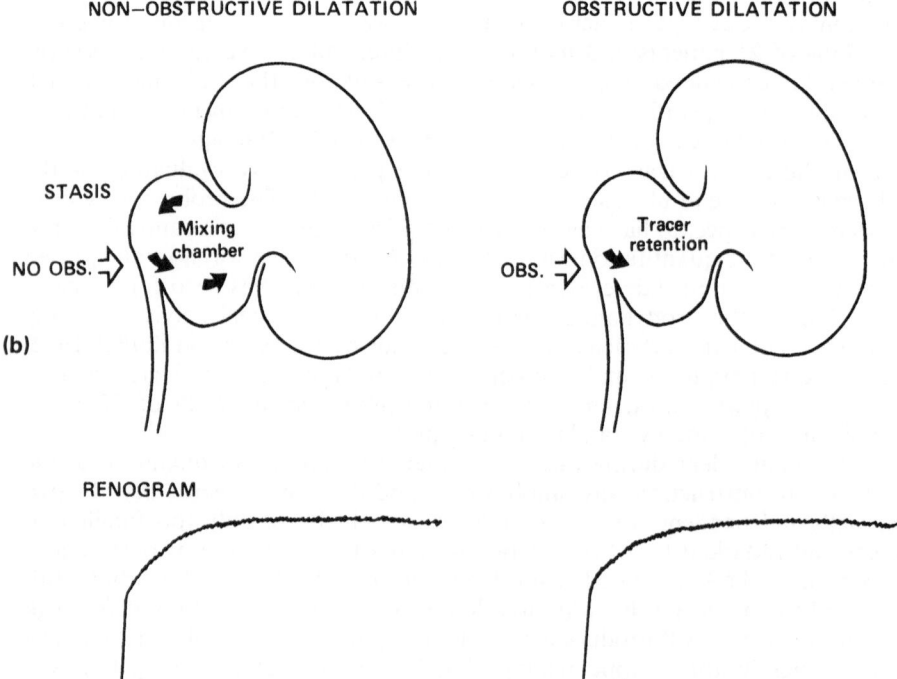

Fig. 4.1a x The normal standard renogram pattern. y The obstructive pattern: **4.1b** identical obstructive renogram patterns caused by stasis in non-obstructive dilatation, and tracer retention in true obstructive dilatation.

Parenchymal Transit Time Studies

Method

Gamma camera renography with ^{123}I-hippuran or ^{99m}Tc-DTPA is performed with the normally hydrated patient sitting in front of the gamma camera. Images are stored in an on-line digital computer system at 20-s intervals for 20–30 min. The images are then summed to allow definition of the whole kidney. Later frames enable the pelvicalyceal system to be identified. Areas of interest are mapped with a light pen over the whole kidney, renal pelvis, bladder, and a vascular region. Activity/time curves are then derived for these regions and the curve for the renal pelvis subtracted from that for the whole kidney to give the parenchymal tracing. Deconvolution analysis of the whole kidney and parenchymal renograms with reference to the vascular curve is then performed.

Deconvolution

The application of deconvolution to the renogram produces a curve called a retention function (Fig. 4.2). The retention function may be regarded as the renogram which would be obtained after an ideal bolus injection directly into the renal artery. There is no recirculation of the tracer and a correction is made for background activity. A sudden rapid initial rise in the curve represents tracer appearance in the kidney; the flat part of the recording corresponds to radionuclide transit through the kidney. In the normal kidney a steep fall in the curve is evident as the tracer disappears from the renal substance. By removing the effects on the renogram of radionuclide recirculation as well as simulating an injection so rapid as

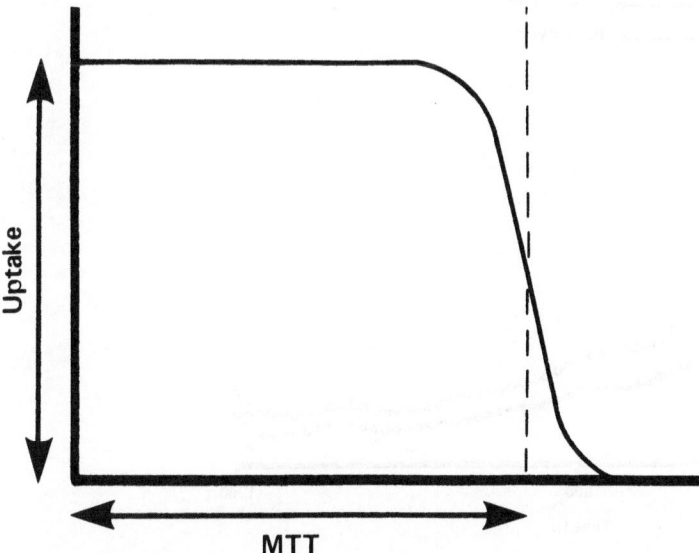

Fig. 4.2. Retention function (MTT, mean transit time).

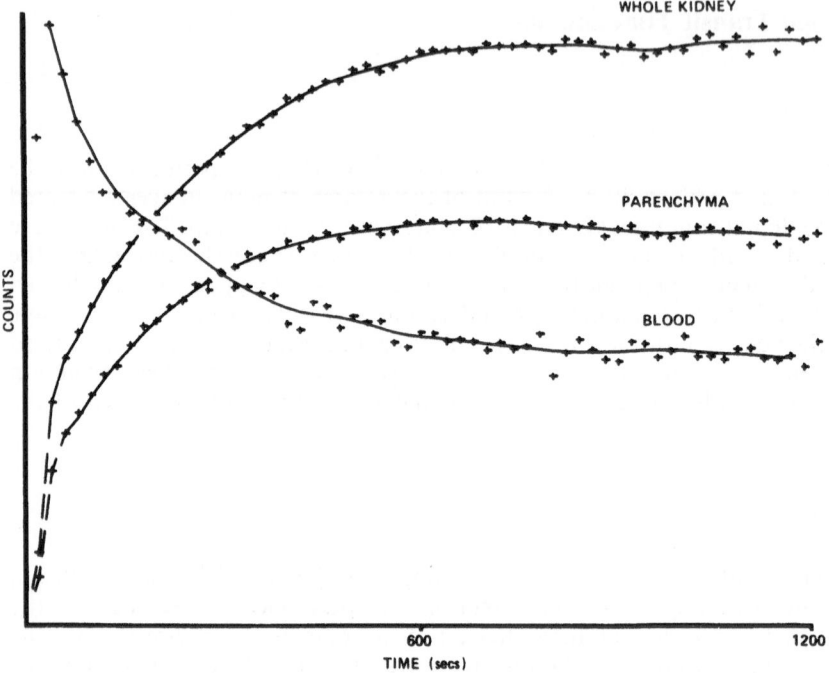

Fig. 4.3. Gamma camera renogram curves from whole kidney and parenchyma in genuine pelviureteric junction obstruction.

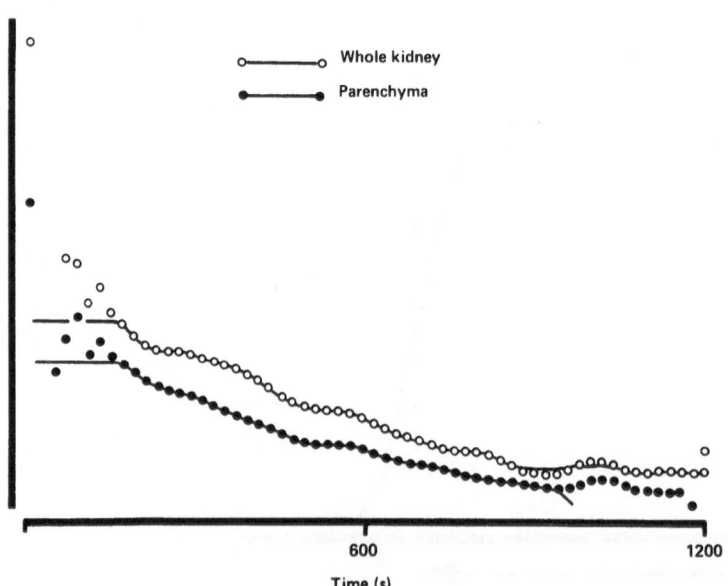

Fig. 4.4. Retention functions from case shown in Fig. 4.3 showing prolonged transit through parenchyma and whole kidney.

to produce no spread of the tracer bolus and correcting for background activity, the retention function allows an effective calculation of various numerical factors relating to renal transit of the tracer and kidney function. These include the minimum transit time, the spread of transit times and the mean transit time. All of these values can be calculated not only for the whole kidney but also for the renal parenchyma alone. For our studies the unmodified mean transit time is the measurement used. Other authors have attempted a correction of this value for the effects of different rates of urine flow—the minimum transit time has been subtracted from the mean transit time to give a transit time index (Whitfield et al. 1977). However, a multicentre combined study on these various parameters of renal function has shown that, while the mean transit time is a reliable and reproducible measurement, the determination of minimum transit time may not be so reliable (Lawson et al. 1979).

The derivation of a renogram over the parenchyma separately from the renal pelvis is occasionally problematical. For example, a thin cortex may not easily be defined separately from a large dilated pelvicalyceal system. The normal 'scatter' of radioactivity from the calyces will have an even greater effect on the parenchymal renogram. Another situation where the parenchymal and pelvic tracings reflect overlap between regions is when the pelvis is mostly intrarenal. Despite these problems it is normally possible to define a 'pure' parenchymal area. An elegant method of distinguishing between pelvis and parenchyma is by the use of a computer algorithm, as described by Whitfield et al. (1978).

Clinical Applications

The derived gamma camera renogram curves for a patient with a kidney obstructed at the pelviureteric junction are shown in Fig. 4.3. The whole kidney renogram has an absent third phase and there is sluggish tracer elimination from the parenchyma. The solid line for each curve shows the data after the smoothing necessary for deconvolution. Figure 4.4 shows the retention functions obtained by deconvoluting the blood curve with the whole kidney and parenchymal renograms. The first few points include non-renal background activity which is subtracted by extrapolating the plateau of each curve back to the origin. The transit of the radiopharmaceutical through both the whole kidney and parenchymal regions is prolonged and the mean transit times are therefore higher than normal. The prolonged parenchymal transit suggests an obstruction which is interfering with renal function. These results are typical of the findings in patients with an obstructive idiopathic hydronephrosis.

The derived renograms for a patient with a non-obstructed, dilated renal pelvis are shown in Fig. 4.5. There is a slow decline of the third phase of the whole kidney renogram but the parenchymal curve is normal in shape. The retention functions obtained by deconvolution analysis of these renograms are shown in Fig. 4.6. The whole kidney mean transit time is prolonged because of stasis of the radiopharmaceutical in the capacious renal pelvis. The parenchymal mean transit time is however normal indicating that the renal pelvic dilatation has not interfered with kidney function. These features are typical of the findings in patients with a non-obstructive idiopathic hydronephrosis.

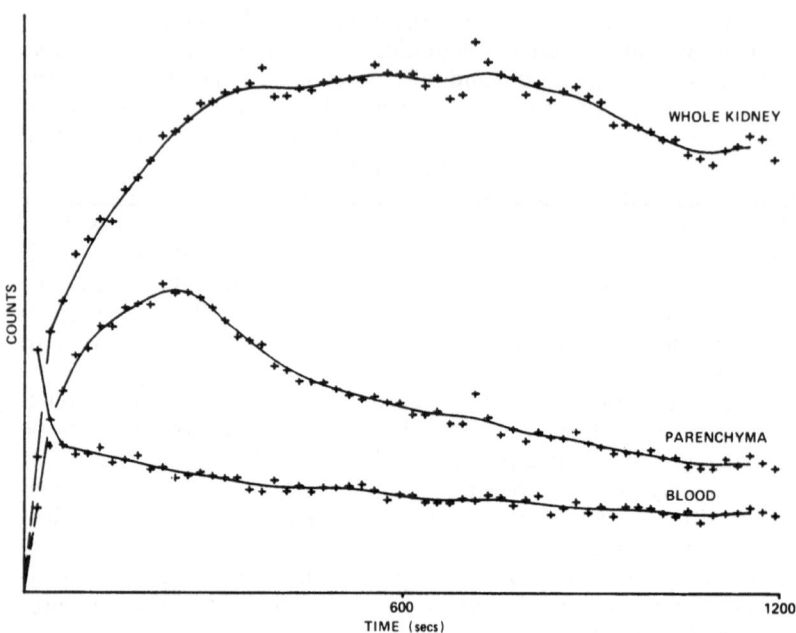

Fig. 4.5. Gamma camera renogram curves from whole kidney and parenchyma in case of non-obstructed dilatation of renal pelvis.

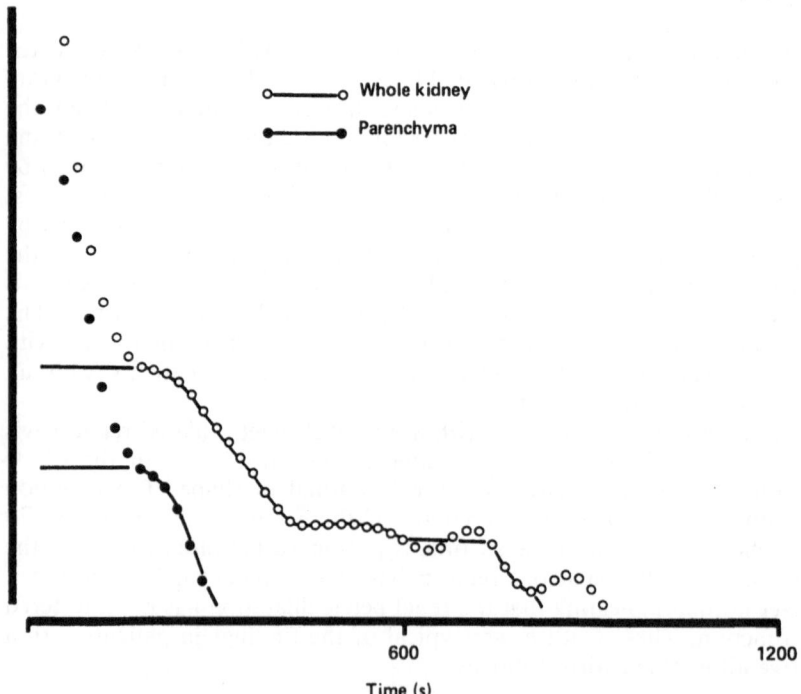

Fig. 4.6. Retention functions from case shown in Fig. 4.5 showing prolonged transit through whole kidney but normal transit through parenchyma.

Diuresis Renography

Method

For preference, ^{123}I-hippuran, or ^{99m}Tc-DTPA, is used for performance of a standard renogram. Thereafter one of three modifications is employed:

a) If the standard renogram is normal, it is repeated 3 min after the intravenous injection of 0.5 mg/kg of the diuretic, frusemide.
b) If the standard renogram shows no elimination at 20 min, the frusemide is given in continuity while the tracing continues uninterrupted.
c) If the standard renogram shows slow spontaneous elimination at 20 min, the frusemide is given in continuity. However, the test should be repeated with the diuretic given from the start if difficulty is experienced in interpreting the curve.

The various responses to the increased flow are shown in Fig. 4.7. In brief:

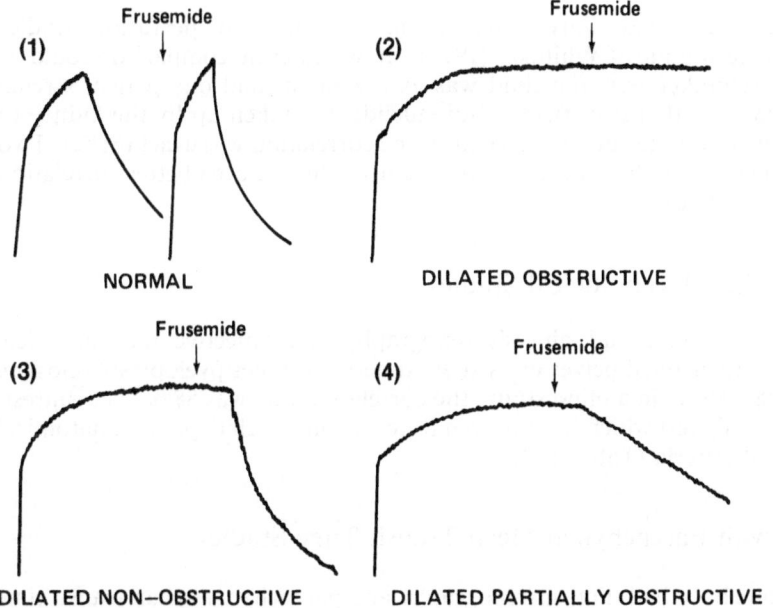

Fig. 4.7.   Diuresis renogram responses in hydronephrosis. (1) normal; (2) dilated obstructed; (3) dilated non-obstructed; (4) dilated partially obstructed.

1) Both renograms may be normal, excluding obstruction.
2) The renogram may be obstructive and remain so after administration of the diuretic, indicating genuine obstructive dilatation.
3) The obstructive curve may revert to normal under diuresis, with rapid, prompt and complete elimination of tracer, indicating a dilated, non-obstructive renal pelvis.
4) The obstructive curve may show a partial elimination response to the diuretic, but not as dramatic as the former response, indicating a sub-total degree of genuine obstruction partially overcome by the increased flow.

It must be emphasised that these responses are but one part of the test, designed to investigate the urodynamics of the system. Of equal importance is the second phase or functional part of the curve, for this is a measure of individual effective renal plasma flow (or GFR if DTPA is used). With the gamma camera, a 2-min hippuran uptake ratio is obtained, the divided function on each side being expressed as a percentage of the total function. This has been shown to correlate well with constant hippuran infusion clearances, renal pelvic urine sampling, and other radionuclide measures of differential function (Hayes et al. 1974; Holter and Storm 1979). The diuresis renogram as described here is the only available procedure which will simultaneously demonstrate renal function and urodynamics.

Since the original description (O'Reilly et al. 1978, 1979), over 350 diuresis renograms have been performed in Manchester alone. There have been no adverse effects in children or adults. The technique has also been compared with the other available means of investigation.

Comparison with Perfusion Studies

Fifteen patients have had diuresis renography followed by perfusion studies according to the technique of Whitaker (1973). In two cases no comparison could be made—in one Whitaker test, the fluid was extravasated, and one patient's renal function was so poor that insufficient radionuclide was taken up by the kidney to allow any comment on the curves. In 11 cases the correlation was exact (85%). Two cases disagreed (15%). Other authors have recently achieved even better correlation (Koff et al. 1979, 1980).

Comparison with Morphological Studies

Forty one patients have had diuresis renography and objective morphological examinations of their renal pelves excised at Anderson–Hynes pyeloplasty (Gosling and Dixon 1978). Here, in a blind study, the correlation rate was 88%. The diuresis renogram is the only test which has yet been tested against such objective anatomical and pathological criteria (Table 4.1).

Comparison with Parenchymal Mean Transit Time Studies

Forty six patients have had diuresis renography and parenchymal mean transit time studies according to the technique of Whitfield et al. (1978) (*vide infra*).

Clinical Applications

It is now policy in our centre to operate on those cases showing the dilated obstructive result and to follow conservatively those showing the dilated non-obstructive pattern. In a recent study of the progress of the latter group, 28 patients were followed up for a period of 1–5 years (O'Reilly et al. to be published). Twenty five had been referred because of unilateral loin pain, two with lower tract symptoms and one with non-specific colicky abdominal pain. All had shown dilatation of the renal pelvis on urography suggestive of possible obstruction (Fig. 4.8). Two renogram patterns were obtained in this group—either a sluggish

Table 4.1. Correlation between diuresis renography and objective renal pelvic morphology

Diuresis renography		Morphology	
		Abnormal	Normal
Dilated obstructed	25	22 (+1 squamous metaplasia)	2
Dilated non-obstructed	8	1	7
Poor function	5	5	–
Equivocal	3	2	1

elimination phase which reverted to normal when the test was repeated under diuresis, or a classic dilated non-obstructed response (Fig. 4.9). Of the 28 patients, 25 (89%) became asymptomatic with conservative management within 12 months of presentation. Their follow-up renograms showed no deterioration in function on urodynamic evaluation. One patient remained symptomatic and developed an equivocal renogram. It was not possible to perform perfusion studies and she had a pyeloplasty. Her post-operative renogram was normal. One patient developed two asymptomatic renal stones but no deterioration in function or elimination. The final patient suffered a transient deterioration in function only, which later returned.

Without the means of objective assessment, most of these patients would probably have proceeded to perhaps well-executed, but totally unnecessary

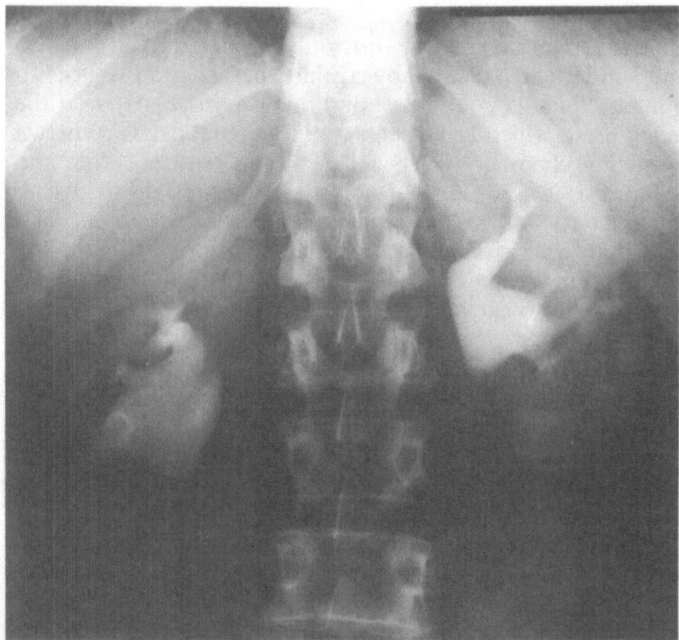

Fig. 4.8. IVU showing dilated renal pelves with no ureteric filling; interpreted as possible due to PUJ obstruction but subsequently shown to be non-obstructed dilatation.

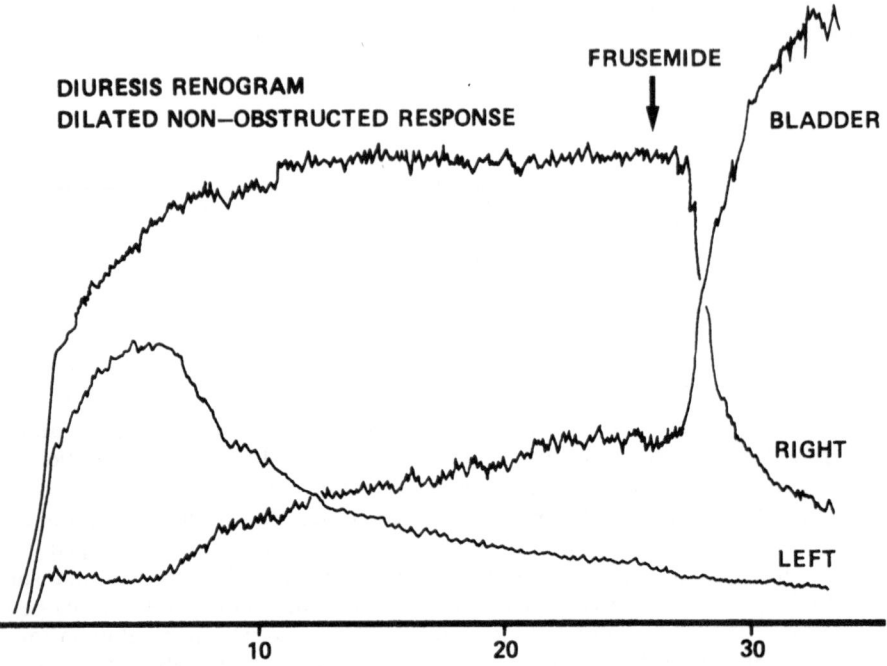

Fig. 4.9. The classic dilated non-obstructed diuresis renogram.

operations, since only one of the 28 ever showed any objective evidence of obstruction.

Current use of the diuresis renogram includes not only pre-operative, but also post-operative evaluation. Sunderland (1963) showed that the urogram returns to normal after pyeloplasty in less than 25% of cases, and this is particularly so if the Culp or Foley techniques are used, which leave behind a large renal pelvis. Where a large pelvis remains, the mixing chamber effect will persist in both urogram and standard renogram unless diuresis is used. Furthermore the urogram fails to give an accurate representation of function— other than to show its presence or absence. (It must be added, however, that where the renogram demonstrates a continuing deterioration in function, the urogram may usefully provide information on parenchymal morphology and help to exclude stone formation.) A recent study of diuresis renography before and after pyeloplasty (Lupton et al. 1979) demonstrated an 88.9% improvement following surgery, compared with only a 50% radiological improvement and 33% improvement in standard renography.

The most common response in this post-surgery group is the dilated non-obstructive pattern. But what produces this pattern? Experimental work has shown that peristalsis may be ineffective in the normal renal pelvis at low flow rates, and in a dilated system, even normal flow rates may be insufficient to allow propagation of the peristaltic wave as far as the ureter. This insufficiency may allow dilatation to persist and stasis to occur. In the obstructed system, this effect is probably compounded by dyssynergia at the pelviureteric junction. What the various pyeloplasty procedures achieve is removal of this dyssynergic segment and, in the Anderson–Hynes technique at least, reduction in the pelvic capacity, thereby allowing urine to reach a wide funnel-shaped proximal ureter. The increased flow through the diuresed non-obstructed kidney has several effects. It will produce an increase in nephron throughput and hydrostatic pressure and enhance effective calyceal pacing and peristalsis thus allowing prompt washout through the non-obstructed PUJ. The theory that this response is produced only in the presence of a high resting pressure and at the expense of a further pressure rise (by implication a damaging pressure rise) is unfounded. In the post-pyeloplasty pelvis, the system is clearly a low pressure one, or by definition the operation has failed. This response is identical in the post-operative case and the new patient with a dilated non-obstructed pelvis. In contrast the situation where excretion *is* produced by diuresis under high pressures occurs in the partially obstructed response discussed earlier. It is not necessary to quantify such cases in terms of pressure— partial renogram obstruction is exactly what it says— partial obstruction requiring active management (Fig. 4.10).

Comparison of Parenchymal Mean Transit Time with Diuresis Renography

The results of these two radionuclide techniques have been compared in 55 kidneys (43 patients) with radiologically demonstrated renal pelvic dilatation. Diuresis renograms were performed and interpreted as described above. The transit times were assessed from gamma camera studies performed on separate occasions. In the 43 patients with suspected idiopathic hydronephrosis the whole kidney mean transit time was prolonged because of tracer retention in the dilated renal pelvis. The important comparison was therefore between the results of diuresis renography and the parenchymal mean transit time since the latter value provides an indication of the effects of renal pelvic dilatation on parenchymal function and transit of the tracer.

A normal range of transit time values were established in 16 kidneys assessed in eight normal volunteers (Table 4.2). The upper limit of normal for parenchymal mean transit time, based on a calculation of two standard deviations above the mean was 239 s.

The ranges, mean values, and standard deviations of the parenchymal mean transit times for kidneys in each of the diuresis renogram groups are shown in Table 4.3. All of the six kidneys with a severe obstruction to urine flow had prolonged parenchymal mean transit times. Of the 11 kidneys with partially obstructive diuresis renograms, eight had higher than normal parenchymal mean transit times. In the other three kidneys (three patients) there was normal parenchymal transit of the tracer. Of these patients two have been managed conservatively; a third has had a pyeloplasty, and pressure/flow studies performed pre-operatively demonstrated an obstructed renal pelvis. There were 29 kidneys with a non-obstructive pattern on

Table 4.2. Parenchymal mean transit time (s) in 16 normal kidneys (8 volunteers)

Mean	169
Range	126–228
Standard deviation	35

Table 4.3. Comparison of parenchymal mean transit times and diuresis renography

	Parenchymal mean transit time (s)		
Diuresis renogram response	Mean	Range	SD
Obstructed (6 kidneys)	470	267–704	152
Partially obstructed (11 kidneys)	297	178–442	92
Non-obstructed (29 kidneys)	212	129–375	57

diuresis renography. In 22 of these cases the parenchymal mean transit time was within normal limits. In seven kidneys, however, the parenchymal transit time was prolonged. (There was a possible explanation for this discrepancy in four cases— one had previously had a renal pelvic operation, another was believed on radiological review to be affected by chronic pyelonephritis and two more kidneys had calculi in the pelvicalyceal systems. It is possible that in these cases there was pelvicalyceal dilatation with impairment of parenchymal function in the absence of obstruction.)

This comparative study between parenchymal transit times and diuresis renography was undertaken since both these radionuclide techniques have been thought to identify those patients with renal pelvic dilatation who are likely to benefit from surgery. Summarising the results, there is a 78% correlation between these two methods of assessment when employed on kidneys with equivocal obstruction. It is likely, however, that the diuresis renogram, in demonstrating the emptying characteristics of the renal pelvis, in addition to giving data on the renal function, is a more specific test for obstruction than parenchymal retention

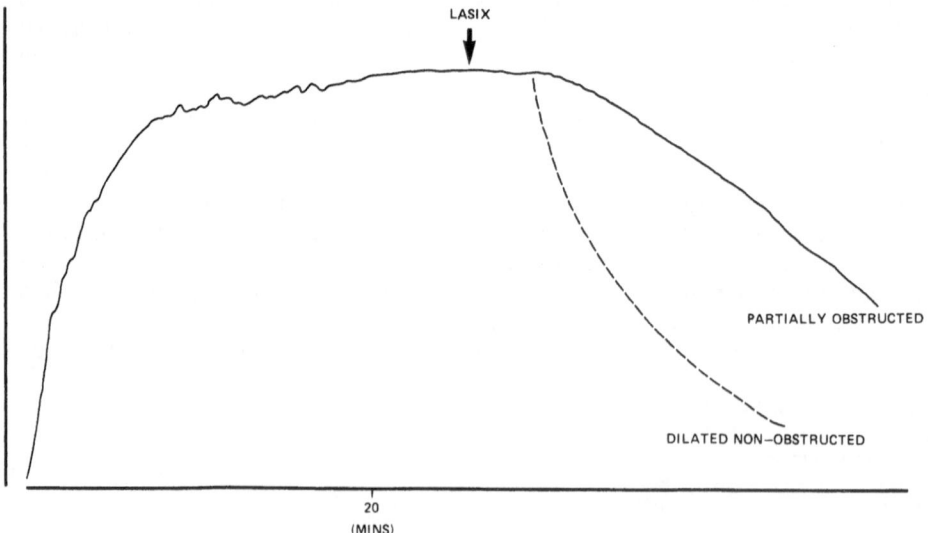

Fig. 4.10. Partially obstructed diuresis renogram response (*dotted line* shows dilated non-obstructed response). Elimination is stimulated, but is slow and inefficient. This response is abnormal and reflects a subtotal impedance to flow.

functions. The latter have the possible disadvantage of being abnormal in disorders in which there is parenchymal functional impairment associated with pelvicalyceal dilatation not caused by obstruction. Both of these investigations have, nevertheless, contributed considerably to the non-invasive assessment of the urographically dilated renal pelvis.

References

Davies RJ, Jones DJ, Croft DN (1969) An assessment of the Anderson–Hynes pyeloplasty by radioisotope renography. Proc R Soc Med 62: 1123-1124

Gosling JA, Dixon JS (1978) Functional obstruction of the upper urinary tract. A histochemical and electron microscopic study. Br J Urol 50: 145-153

Hayes M, Brosnan S, Taplin GV (1974) Determination of differential renal function by sequential scintography. J Urol 111: 556-559

Holten I, Storm HH (1979) Kidney scintography with ^{99}Tc-DMSA and ^{131}I-hippuran. Scand J Urol Nephrol 131: 275-283

Johnston JH, Kathel BL (1972) The results of surgery for hydronephrosis as determined by isotope renography with analogue computer simulation. Br J Urol 44: 320-327

Karlberg I (1976) Hydronephrosis: An assessment of late results of treatment of pelviureteric junction obstruction. Scand J Urol Nephrol 10: 235-238

Koff SA, Thrall JH, Keyes JW Jr (1979) Diuretic radionuclide urography: A non-invasive method for evaluating nephroureteral dilation. J Urol 122: 451-454

Koff SA, Thrall JH, Keyes JW Jr (1980) Assessment of hydroureteronephrosis in children using diuretic radionuclide urography. J Urol 123: 531-534

Lawson RS, Brown NGJ, Dance DR, Diffey BL, Erbsmann F, Fleming JS, Houston AS, Tofts PS (1979) A multicentre comparison of techniques for deconvolution of the renogram. Communication to the British Nuclear Medicine Society, Seventh Annual Meeting, April 1979

Lupton EW, Testa HJ, Lawson RS, Charlton-Edwards E, Carroll RNP, Barnard RJ (1979) Diuresis renography and the results of pyeloplasty for idiopathic hydronephrosis. Br J Urol 51: 449-453

O'Reilly PH, Testa HJ, Lawson RS, Farrar DJ, Charlton-Edwards E (1978) Diuresis renography in equivocal urinary tract obstruction. Br J Urol 50: 76-80

O'Reilly PH, Lawson RS, Shields RA, Testa HJ (1979) Idiopathic hydronephrosis. J Urol 121: 153-155

O'Reilly PH, Lupton EW, Shields RA, Testa HJ, Carroll RNP and Charlton-Edwards E (to be published) The dilated non-obstructed renal pelvis. Br J Urol

Otnes B, Rootwelt K, Mathison W (1975) A comparison between urography and isotope renography in the follow up of surgery for hydronephrosis. Scand J Urol Nephrol 9: 50-56

Roberts M, Slade N, Jeffery P (1972) Late results in the management of primary pelvic hydronephrosis. Br J Urol 44: 15-18

Sunderland H (1963) A review of experience with the Anderson–Hynes plastic operation for hydronephrosis. Br J Urol 35: 1

Taplin GV, Meredith OM, Kade H, Winter CC (1956) The radioisotope renogram. J Lab Clin Med 48: 886

Tveter KS, Nerdrum HJ, Mjolnerod OK (1975) The value of radioisotope renography in the follow-up of patients operated on for hydronephrosis. J Urol 47: 781-787

Whitaker RH (1973) Diagnosis of obstruction in dilated ureters. Ann R Coll Surg Engl 53: 153-166

Whitfield HN, Britton KE, Kelsey Fry I, Hendry WF, Nimmon CC, Travers P, Wickham JEA (1977) The obstructed kidney: Correlation between renal function and urodynamic assessment. Br J Urol 49: 615-619

Whitfield HN, Britton KE, Hendry WF, Nimmon CC, Wickham JEA (1978) The distinction between obstructive uropathy and nephropathy by radioisotope transit times. Br J Urol 50: 433-436

5. Pressure Flow Studies I

R.H. Whitaker

It was always believed and stated in the urological literature that 'dilated' urinary tracts were obstructed. Indeed, until the significance of vesicoureteric reflux was appreciated the words *dilated* and *obstructed* were almost synonymous. This attitude is reflected in the early classifications of megaureters where two types were described— refluxing and obstructed. It was Shopfner (1966) who suggested that perhaps not all wide or dilated systems were truly obstructed, but it has taken many more years for this message to be appreciated. The first proof that he was correct was provided by Backlund and Reuterskiöld (1969), who were able to demonstrate low pressures on perfusion in some dilated systems showing the absence of obstruction.

This dynamic evaluation was taken up by Johnston (1969), who studied hydronephrosis in a similar way and stressed that hydronephrosis is not an 'all-or-none' phenomenon. Early efforts to define obstruction (Whitaker 1973c) in meaningful and clinically applicable terms laid even more emphasis on the dynamic aspects of obstruction— *a narrowing such that the proximal pressure is raised to transmit the usual flow through it.* Thus, in the early stages of our investigations of obstruction, as defined above, it seemed that the most logical approach was to measure the pressures and flows and try to define the limits of resistance of normal and abnormal urinary tracts. Some early studies (Whitaker 1973b) simply measured the pressure in the renal pelvis during a diuresis, but the results were difficult to interpret as the diuresis was often of unknown quantity and although a high pressure was meaningful a low pressure did not exclude an obstruction. The idea of perfusing into the system was then introduced so that a known flow rate was established and the pressures could be interpreted as a definite relationship to it. These early experiments led to the development of a clinical test that was first described in 1973 (Whitaker 1973a).

Clinical Application

The main advantage of this test over other previous attempts at studying the upper urinary tract dynamically is that a single cannula is introduced percutaneously and through it fluid is perfused and the pressure measured.

Technique

Following an explanation of the procedure, the patient is premedicated with Valium orally an hour before, or intravenously at the time of the procedure. In younger children a general anaesthetic is needed, but this is quite unnecessary in older patients. The procedure is performed in the X-ray department with full screening facilities. Initially the patient lies supine so that intravenous contrast medium can be given to demonstrate the urinary tract and also so that a small urethral catheter can be inserted into the bladder. In children an infant feeding tube is employed. If the problem is an equivocal pelviureteric junction obstruction then the bladder is emptied. If there is any question of a secondary dilatation of the upper urinary tract the bladder can be left full for the initial part of the investigation. The bladder pressure is recorded via a 20-cm manometer tube and stopcock using a single transducer (Fig. 5.1).

The patient is then turned prone so that the kidney in question is nearest to the investigator. A small pillow under the abdomen is useful to push the kidneys gently backwards. Intermittent screening indicates when contrast medium has reached the pelvicalyceal system and a mark on the skin shows the site for puncture (Fig. 5.2). The skin and deeper tissues are infiltrated with local anaesthetic and a 4- or 6-in. 18G Longdwel cannula is introduced vertically downwards into the collecting system. Full details of the technique have been described elsewhere (Whitaker 1979b). The equipment is minimal, as shown in Figs. 5.2 and 5.3.

All major departments of radiology probably have radiologists who are adept at pelvicalyceal puncture and further details of this standard technique are not required. The cannula is adjusted so that the perfusion can run freely either via a calix, or via the renal pelvis. Screening allows detection of leaks of the contrast medium, which occasionally occur. For perfusion, 30% Urografin, or similar medium is used and the rate used initially is 10 ml/min. Despite some criticism this rate is well within the physiological range. Furthermore the object of the test is to stress the system to produce the maximal pressure so that the slightest sign of obstruction can be detected. Intermittent screening during the procedure together with spot films allows good visualisation of the anatomy and behaviour of the upper tract.

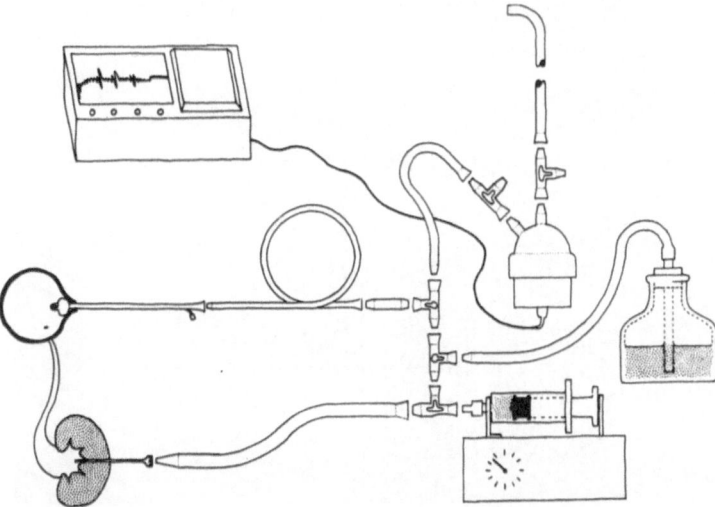

Fig. 5.1. The various connections of the equipment used for pressure flow studies. Adapted from Urologic Clinics of North America 1979, 6: 533, by kind permission of the publishers.

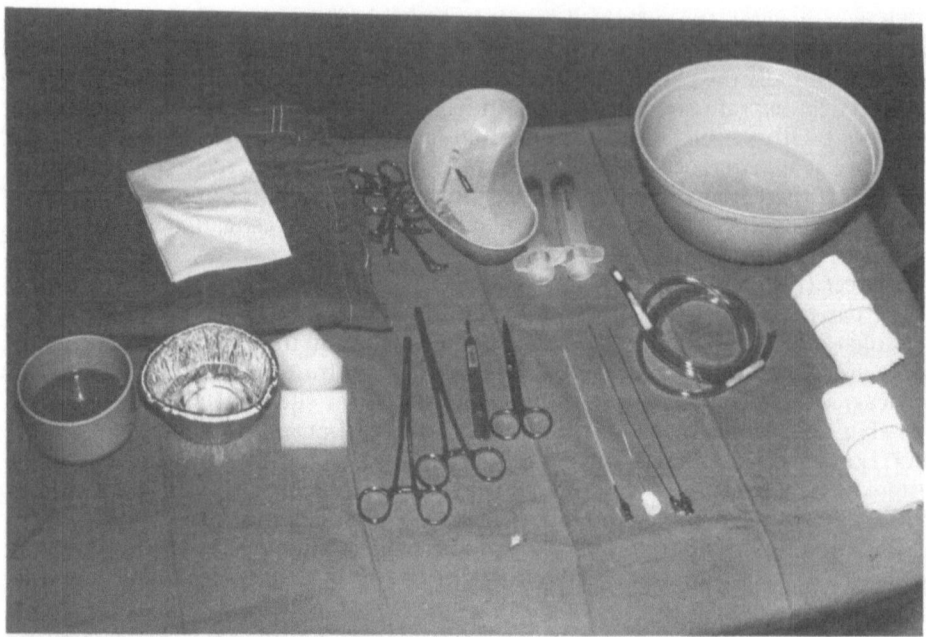

Fig. 5.2. Equipment needed for percutaneous antegrade puncture of the kidney. From Urologic Clinics of North America 1979, 6: 534, by kind permission of the publishers.

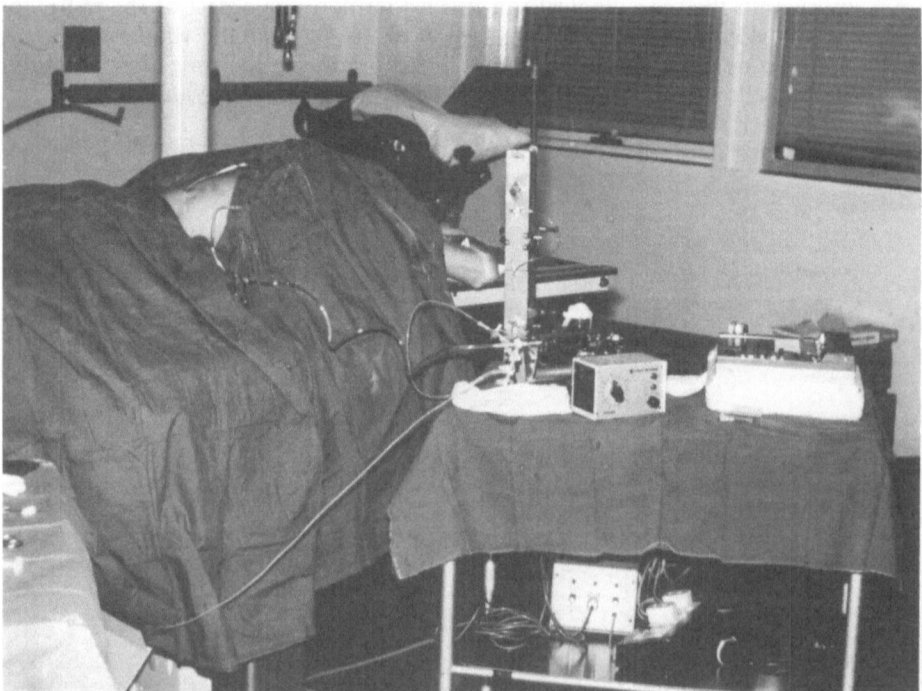

Fig. 5.3. Patient lying prone during a study with the kidney under investigation nearest to the operator. The bladder pressure line is seen passing under the sheet. From Urologic Clinics of North America 1979, 6: 532, by kind permission of the publishers.

The bladder is allowed to fill and its pressure is measured by intermittently opening the stopcock connected to the transducer. It is essential to continue the perfusion until the system is equilibrated— i.e. the flow into the kidney is the same as the flow into the bladder. Only then should the final pressure reading within the kidney be taken. After the procedure the fluid within the kidney is aspirated and the cannula removed. The cannula is then perfused in air at the same rate to estimate its intrinsic resistance. This figure is needed to calculate the final result. The patient is kept in bed for 12 h with regular monitoring of blood pressure and pulse.

Complications

As with any renal puncture haematuria is to be expected, but this has only once, in our experience, led to clot colic and some distress. Blood transfusion has not been required in any patient but one urinary tract infection was attributable to the study. In general the study is well tolerated in patients and its minor discomfort is less than the after-effects of a short anaesthetic.

Interpretation of Results

In assessing the results it should be remembered that the principle is simply to detect an abnormally high pressure during a simulated diuresis as an indication of obstruction. Furthermore, it is the nephrons that are adversely affected by the raised pressure so that it is the pressure within the renal pelvis that is of particular concern. If it is assumed for the sake of the present discussion on hydronephrosis that the bladder pressures are normal then the bladder pressure can be subtracted from the renal pelvic pressure to give a measure of the pressure drop across the suspected site of obstruction— in this case the pelviureteric junction. The resistance of the cannula (the pressure it generates to perfusion of 10 ml/min) must also be subtracted to give the final relative pressure.

It is not clear from experimental studies on animals as to what level of pressure is needed to cause renal damage, or indeed how long such pressure needs to be applied. However, after an experience of over 200 pressure measurements in humans (and supported by the work of Schweitzer (1973) who showed that renal function was easily affected by pressure), it is considered that a pressure of 15 cmH$_2$O at 10 ml/min probably represents the upper limit of normal: pressures of 22 cmH$_2$O and above indicate an obstruction which requires surgical intervention.

Indications in Equivocal Hydronephrosis

Despite the very real advances in isotope assessment of upper urinary tract obstruction an important place for dynamic assessment still exists. The information that the antegrade pyelogram provides in terms of anatomy and pathophysiology, together with accurate and comparable pressure measurement has encouraged us to continue to use the pressure flow technique as the definite method. The results of diuresis renography are equivocal in some cases and may suggest, but not confirm a partial obstruction. The pressure flow method can quantitate such obstruction if it exists. Furthermore, parenchymal transit times are technically difficult, particularly in kidneys with a thin parenchyma.

An additional problem in hydronephrosis concerns intermittent obstruction since none of the above tests demonstrate latent obstruction. In these patients we have found that only a urogram at the time of pain provides the diagnosis (Chap. 3).

Over the years conventional means of assessment of obstruction in these equivocal patients have proved unreliable as shown by later dynamic studies. Thus, urography and ureterography in conjunction with non-diuretic renography must be interpreted with great caution.

To those who believe that they cannot afford the time to study a patient with such an equivocal problem for an hour or so (or that they have not the equipment), it should be borne in mind that it is better to spend an hour making the correct diagnosis than to offer the patient an unnecessary and perhaps hazardous operation. There seems little doubt that many unnecessary pyeloplasties have been performed over the years throughout the world, and it seems likely that some of these have left the patients worse off than before the operation. It now behoves the urologist to look more carefully at these equivocal cases and be sure whether or not there is a real evidence of obstruction.

Cystography should be performed if there is any question at all of vesicoureteric reflux as some types of pelviureteric junction obstruction can be precipitated by the reflux itself (Whitaker and Flower 1979).

Results of Pressure Flow Measurement

Over 200 of these studies have now been performed in Cambridge and the results of the first 170 undertaken in 112 patients have recently been analysed (Whitaker 1979a). Of these studies 96% gave either a clear indication of no obstruction (< 12 cmH$_2$O) or showed definite obstruction (> 22 cm H$_2$O) at 10 ml/min. Thus in only 4% of these already equivocal cases was the result uncertain, viz. pressures between 15 and 22 cmH$_2$O.

An analysis of the studies performed in equivocal hydronephrosis in which a pelviureteric obstruction was in doubt has recently been made. Over the last few years 75 patients have been studied. In 40 of these patients the left kidney had equivocal hydronephrosis and in 35 the right kidney was in doubt. Thirty-six patients were found to have no obstruction. In these patients a pressure range of 2-14 cmH$_2$O (average 8 cmH$_2$O) was obtained. Definite evidence of obstruction with pressures between 20 and 100 cmH$_2$O was shown by 39 patients and only one (the patient with a pressure of 20 cmH$_2$O) fell into the so-called equivocal range (15-22 cm H$_2$O). Thus the study gave an unequivocal answer as to whether or not there was obstruction in 74 of 75 cases (98.5%).

In 20 of these 75 cases of equivocal hydronephrosis renography was also performed. This was not done according to the strict criteria of the Manchester group, and it was undoubtedly because of this that only 12 cases showed complete agreement. However, amongst these cases there was one example of what seemed to be a genuine discrepancy between the two methods. It seems that there is still a need for very careful studies comparing these two techniques.

Summary

The most important aspect of equivocal hydronephrosis is to accept that the problem exists and that it needs more investigation than a urogram and ureterogram. Pressure flow studies offer a reliable, albeit invasive method of investigation and only rarely give an equivocal answer. Sophisticated renography often proves valuable, but still leaves some patients in whom the answer is unresolved. A multidisciplinary approach may well prove to be the best approach.

References

Backlund L, Reuterskiold AG (1969) The abnormal ureter in children. I. Perfusion studies on the wide non-refluxing ureter. Scand J Urol Nephrol 3: 219-228

Johnston JH (1969) Pathogenesis of hydronephrosis in children. Br J Urol 41: 724-734

Schweitzer FAW (1973) Intrapelvic pressure and renal function studies in experimental chronic partial ureteric obstruction. Br J Urol 45: 2-7

Shopfner CE (1966) Ureteropelvic junction obstruction. AJR 98: 148-159

Whitaker RH (1973a) Methods of assessing obstruction in dilated ureters. Br J Urol 45: 15-22

Whitaker RH (1973b) Diagnosis of obstruction in dilated ureters. Ann R Coll Surg Engl 53: 153-166

Whitaker RH (1973c) The ureter in posterior urethral valves. Br J Urol 45: 395-403

Whitaker RH (1979a) An evaluation of 170 diagnostic pressure flow studies of the upper urinary tract. Br J Urol 121: 602-604

Whitaker RH (1979b) The Whitaker test. Urol Clin North Am 6: 529-539

Whitaker RH, Flower CDR (1979) Ureters that show both reflux and obstruction. Br J Urol 51: 471-474

6. Pressure Flow Studies II

R.C. Pfister

Since their introduction in 1973, perfusion studies for the assessment of pyeloureteral dynamics have been extensively evaluated at the Massachusetts General Hospital and, as suggested by Whitaker, the technique has proven to be valuable.

Pelviureteric junction (PUJ) obstruction constitutes an important cause of intrarenal dilatation. In some cases the diagnosis is obvious from standard and modified (diuretic) urography and radionuclide studies (Koff et al. 1979, 1980; O'Reilly et al. 1978, 1979; Whitfield et al. 1977). In others the diagnosis of obstruction at the PUJ is questionable or uncertain and pressure flow studies are particularly useful.

This chapter describes the technique for perfusion studies (PFS) used at the Massachusetts General Hospital for the past 6 years (Pfister 1978; Pfister and Newhouse 1978, 1979; Yoder and Pfister 1978).

Technique

Equipment and Recording

A basic list of equipment is provided in Table 6.1. The method, as described by Whitaker (1973, 1975, 1976, 1978, 1979a,b,c) has been significantly modified to minimise renal damage, decrease instrumentation complexity and reduce examination time in a busy clinical practice. Thus, a thin flexible 22g needle for renal perfusion is employed and the pressure transducer and chart recorder are omitted (Fig. 6.1). Since pressure transducers must be calibrated with a simple water manometer at each examination, their use is only justified if a permanent paper recording of renal pelvis and bladder pressures during different flow rate perfusion runs is desired. In our experience, a pen or strip recorder serves no significant purpose and only accumulates reams of paper. In addition, the cost of these items is considerable.

We have chosen to obtain renal and bladder pressures intermittently during each perfusion sequence and immediately record (a) pressure, (b) perfusion rate and time, and (c) bladder volume on a pre-designed perfusion data sheet, which also has columns for noting frequency and percent of coaptation of ureteral peristalsis. Space for a pertinent history and details of the study are provided alongside a drawing of a normal urinary tract which permits heavy solid-line drawing of the current anatomic situation (Fig. 6.2).

Table 6.1. Equipment for perfusion studies

Hardware

   Infusion pump (Sigmamotor; double head, 4004)

   Intravenous stands (2), moveable (6 ft)

   Table, moveable (24 × 36 in.)

Sterile disposables

   Infusion pump tubing (Sigmamotor, 8403)

   Manometers (2), plastic 56 cm (Medex, MX2694: 04170-12)

   Three-way stopcocks (2), plastic (Pharmaseal)

   Thin flexible 22g needle; 4, 9 and 15 cm (Sherwood)

   Urethral catheter, 5 and 10 Fr feeding tube, 15 in. (Angyle)

   168 cm needle extension line (Pharmaseal, K50L)

   168 cm urethral extension line (Pharmaseal, K50L)

   84 cm manometer extension lines (2) (Pharmaseal)

   Diluted (20%) contrast medium bottles (2) (500 ml)

   230 cm positive pressure extension line, bottle (McGaw)

   250ml bowl; urethral catheter (Superior, 610)

PERCUTANEOUS PERFUSION TECHNIQUE

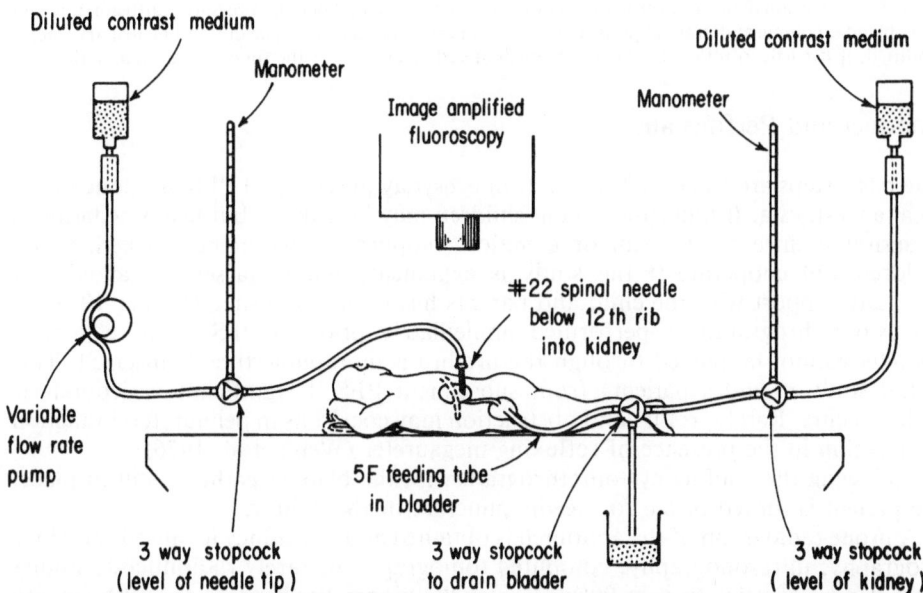

Fig. 6.1. Schematic representation of simplified prone percutaneous ureteral perfusion examination immediately following supine voiding cystourethrography. Disposable water manometers are interfaced with the bladder catheter and 22g renal needle.

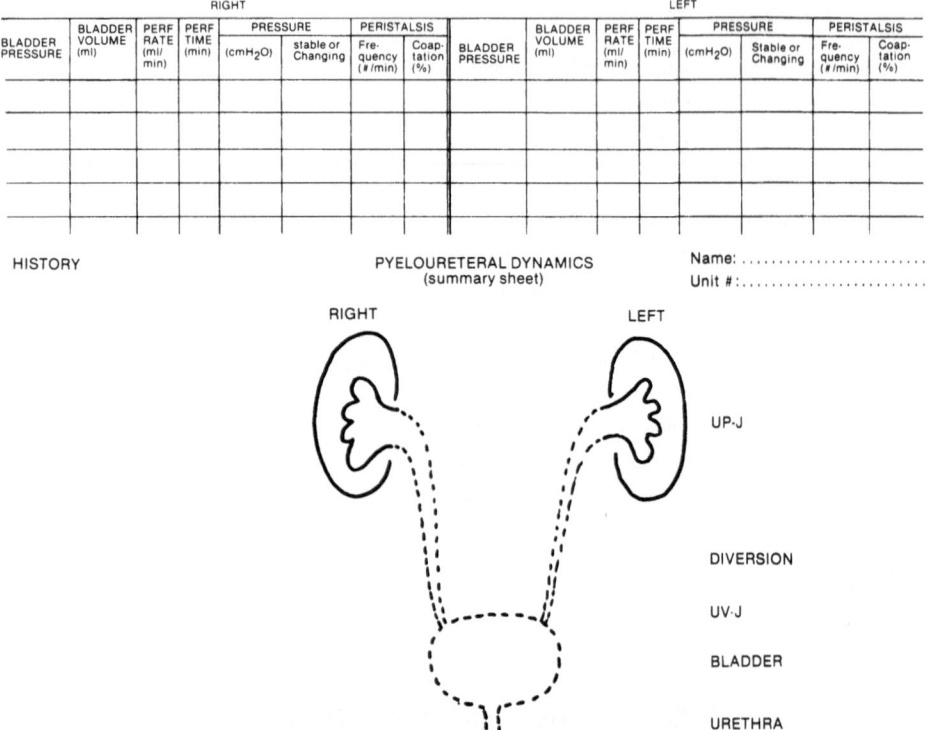

		RIGHT									LEFT							
				PRESSURE		PERISTALSIS							PRESSURE		PERISTALSIS	
BLADDER PRESSURE	BLADDER VOLUME (ml)	PERF RATE (ml/min)	PERF TIME (min)	(cmH₂O)	stable or Changing	Fre-quency (#/min)	Coap-tation (%)	BLADDER PRESSURE	BLADDER VOLUME (ml)	PERF RATE (ml/min)	PERF TIME (min)	(cmH₂O)	Stable or Changing	Fre-quency (#/min)	Coap-tation (%)

HISTORY   PYELOURETERAL DYNAMICS   Name: ....
                              (summary sheet)   Unit #: ....

RIGHT   LEFT

UP-J

DIVERSION

UV-J

BLADDER

URETHRA

Fig. 6.2. Perfusion data sheet for permanent recording of renal and bladder pressures, infusion rate and time, bladder volume and ureteral peristalsis for each perfusion sequence. The dotted-line urinary tract is modified, if needed, to reflect the anatomy encountered or existing at the time of the examination.

Conduct and Performance

The basic steps are listed in Table 6.2. In everyday practice, all PFS are done under local anaesthesia. Infants and young children may be sedated but heavy sedation is undesirable since severe pain or a major complication might be masked. Older children will cooperate if the study is explained, and surprises are avoided if adequate rapport with the child and parents has been established (Pfister 1978).

Cystourethrography is performed immediately prior to PFS. If a retrograde catheter cannot be passed through the urethra a suprapubic tube is inserted. This initial study excludes patients from subsequent PFS if significant vesicoureteric reflux occurs. Rarely, reflux and obstruction may coexist as in pelviureteric junction obstruction in the presence of refluxing megaureter (Weiss et al. 1976).

Following the voiding cystourethrogram with the bladder catheter still in place, the patient is turned prone for needle puncture of the kidney.

A prone radiograph of the abdomen is obtained and the kidney localised; previous urography, ultrasonography, computed tomography or rarely radionuclide studies may also be of help. In over 90% of cases the kidney lies beneath the 12th rib and this site is prepared and draped. If the kidney is very low (as in an ectopic pelvic kidney) an anterior abdominal wall approach is used and the patient remains in a supine position.

Table 6.2. Technique for ureteral perfusion

---

1)   Bladder catheterisation, 6–10 Fr straight tube

2)   Voiding cystourethrography, leaving catheter in place

3)   Antegrade pyelography[a]

      a)   Position patient, 'prep' and drape skin

      b)   Localise kidney

      c)   Inject local anaesthetic agent

      d)   Puncture collecting system, single 22g needle[b]

      e)   Aspirate urine sample

      f)   Measure pressure, check free flow

      g)   Inject contrast medium, fluoroscopic control

      h)   Radiograph (optional)

4)   Ureteral perfusion (empty bladder); intermittent fluoroscopy and pressure recordings (renal and bladder); radiograph

5)   Variable rate perfusion runs (5, 10, 15, 20 ml/min) as desired/needed

6)   Ureteral perfusion (full bladder); remainder of steps 4) and 5)

---

[a]Sedation for infants, young children (mixture of meperidine 25 mg, promethazine 5 mg and chlorpromazine 8 mg. Dose of 1 ml/25 lb but not to exceed 2 ml).

[b]Perfusion and pressure recording can be performed through a single larger-bore needle/catheter. Our experience suggests that two smaller needles cause less haematuria and can be utilised if constant pressure monitoring is desired; also obviates calculation of needle resistance at each flow rate.

Intravenous contrast medium for imaging the kidney during needle puncture has only been used in 1% of cases. When employed, it is used on non-dilated or minimally dilated collecting systems.

In all other instances the palpable 12th rib and fluoroscopically visible landmarks (rib, transverse processes) are used to localise the kidney. With good quality image-intensified fluoroscopy the kidney itself is often visible.

The needle site is anaesthetised with 1% xylocaine. A thin 22g needle of length (4, 9, 15 cm) appropriate to patient size is chosen for puncture.

A 10-ml syringe containing 3–4 ml local anaesthetic is attached to the needle and used for further anaesthesia and for puncture of the pyelocalyceal system. The needle is advanced from a direct posterior (vertical) direction taking care that arching is avoided to prevent false-tracking. Intermittent injections of small amounts of xylocaine during needle advancement prevents plugging of the lumen. An alternating injection–aspiration sequence is used; free urine-return signals successful entry into the pelvicalyceal system. Entry of the needle tip into the posterior renal cortex can be verified fluoroscopically since the needle will flex synchronously with renal respiratory motion. If the appropriate depth has been reached but no urine obtained, the needle is slowly retracted with continuous aspiration to the skin and then readvanced using a slightly different trajectory path. In the usual case one to three needle passes will be required for successful placement.

The first 2–4 ml aspirated urine is retained for culture or other determinations. A saline-flushed water manometer with three-way stopcock and extension tubing are then attached to the needle. Opening or resting pressure is obtained with the zero point of the manometer at the level of the needle tip.

Free flow of fluid through the needle tip is verified by raising and/or lowering the manometer; a fixed pressure indicates absence of free flow and requires adjustment

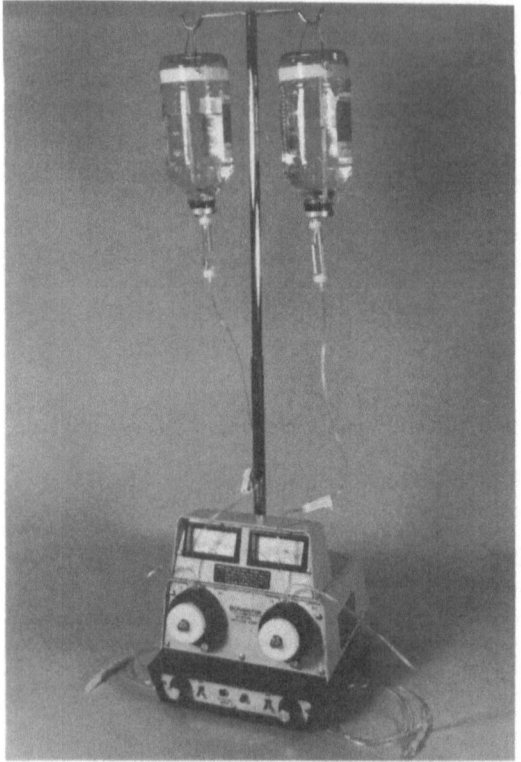

Fig. 6.3. Variable rate (1–20 ml/min) dual-head infusion pump capable of perfusing both kidneys simultaneously at separate rates with diluted contrast medium within the suspended bottles. The pump is stored on a moveable table or cart.

of the needle tip. Injection of contrast medium without readjustment is fruitless since some degree of extravasation outside the pelvicalyceal system will occur.

Once free flow of urine has been obtained contrast medium can be injected under fluoroscopic control and spot films obtained.

Perfusion is performed by a double-head infusion pump. Each head is capable of constant-speed delivery rates of 1-ml increments up to 20 ml/min. We have found that syringe-delivery type pumps are unable to deliver fluid at high flow rates through the small 22g needle employed. Bottles up to 500 ml volume containing the infusion fluid are suspended above each pump head (Fig. 6.3).

The infusion fluid is contrast medium diluted to 20% concentration. We have avoided saline as a perfusate since it is invisible fluoroscopically and on radiographs; extravasation with or without pain is not detectable without opaque contrast medium.

Usually, a flow rate of 5–10 ml/min is initially delivered under intermittent fluoroscopic control with intermittent pressure readings until steady-state perfusion exists. Such steady-state equilibrium is present when the entire upper tract is filled and pressure is unchanging after several minutes of perfusion at a given flow rate (Fig. 6.4).

In the presence of significant obstruction, perfusion time and/or rate of delivery should be lower to avoid excessively high intrapelvic pressures. We have limited

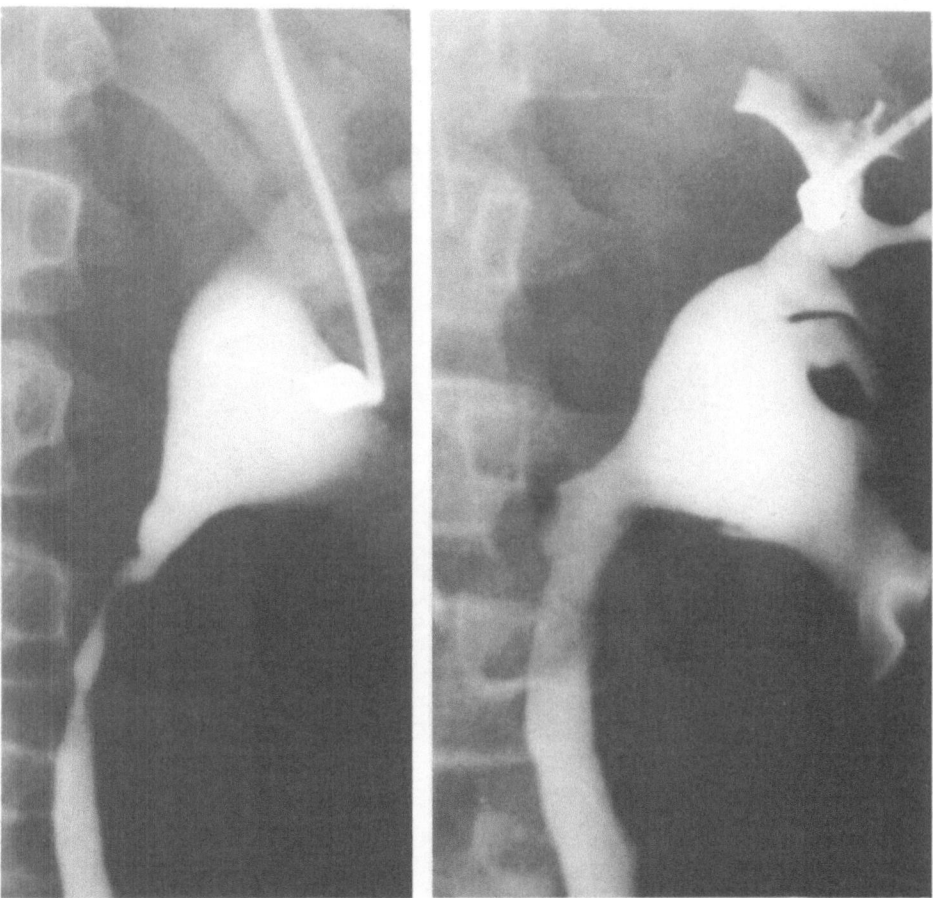

a
b

Fig. 6.4. Eleven-year-old boy some four years post-pyeloplasty elsewhere for congenital PUJ obstruction. **a** Perfusion run at 10 ml/min for 10 min resulted in differential pressure of 12–13 cmH$_2$O with the bladder empty. **b** Repeat perfusion sequence 9 months following second pyeloplasty; differential pressure of 6–7 cmH$_2$O at the same flow rate and similar empty bladder pressure. Note the decrease in the calyectasis besides the obvious anatomic alteration in the PUJ between the two pyeloplasty perfusion studies.

maximal renal pressure during perfusion to 40–50 cmH$_2$O since intrarenal and intravascular reflux may occur with intracalyceal pressures above 30 cmH$_2$O. In markedly dilated upper urinary systems, perfusion time and/or delivery rate need to be increased to reach steady-state perfusion.

Because of the small bore of the renal needle, the viscosity of the infusion fluid and the flow rates employed, the pressure response to perfusion is obtained immediately after the pump is turned off by switching the stopcock on the manometer. By alternatively turning the pump on and off and obtaining intermittent pressures the effect of a given flow rate can be monitored. When satisfied that steady-state response has been obtained at a given flow rate, with the bladder empty and full, the pressure data of the kidney and bladder, the bladder volume, the perfusion time and the effect of peristalsis are entered on the permanent record sheet.

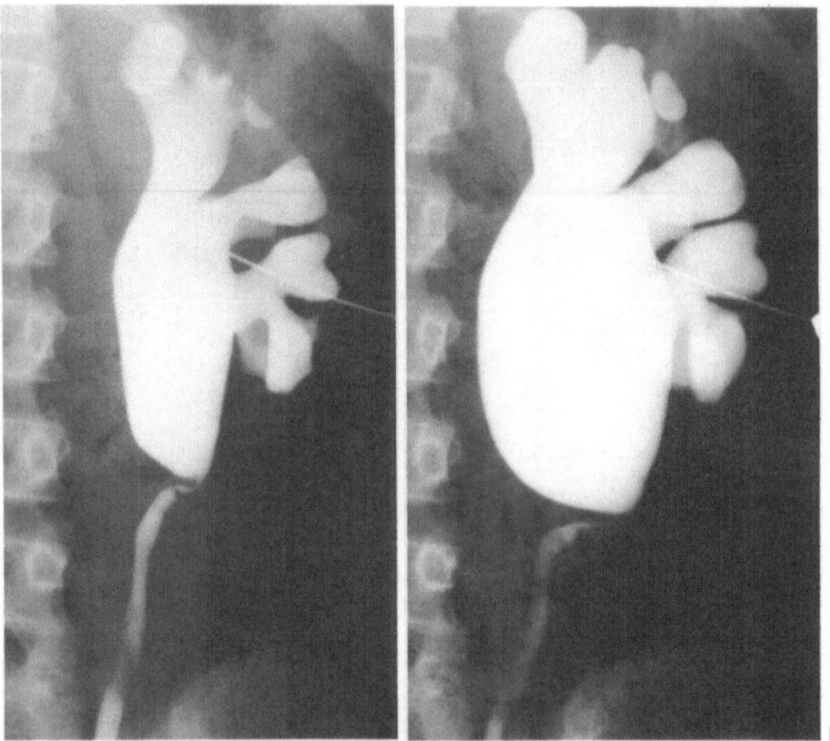

a   b

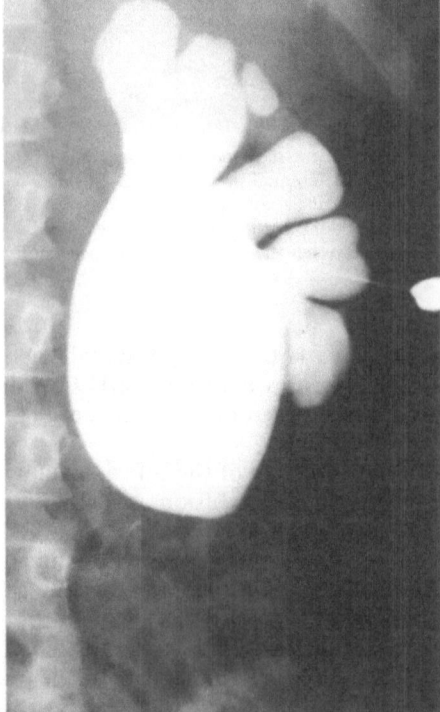

c

Fig. 6.5. Eleven-year-old girl with recurrent left flank pain in recent months. Percutaneous perfusion study at different steady-state flow rates lasting seven minutes for each of the first two runs; empty bladder pressure of 4 cmH$_2$O. **a** 10 ml/min, **b** 15 ml/min and **c** 20 ml/min flow rate sequences resulted in renal pelvis pressures of 14, 18 and 25 cmH$_2$O, respectively. The PUJ decompensated at the highest flow rate and renal pressure rapidly rose reproducing her flank pain; perfusion was stopped and the renal pelvis was aspirated until empty prior to removing the needle. Note that differential pressures of 10, 14 and 21 cmH$_2$O were 'normal', 'equivocal', and 'abnormal', respectively by our standards; perfusion at the standard rate (10 ml/min) would have resulted in a false-negative result.

The interval pressure values obtained by this modification are exactly similar to the data obtained with a constant pressure recorder and large-bore needles or catheters that require pre- or post-perfusion calibration for the pressure drops produced by various flow rates. In addition, the intermittent perfusion-pressure monitoring technique is quick and simple as it does not require the more complex pressure transducer and pen chart or graph recorder.

In equivocal obstruction or when differential pressures are in the 'high normal, indeterminate and low abnormal' ranges the flow rate can be increased from the standard 10 ml/min to 15–20 ml/min (Pfister and Newhouse 1980). The higher flow rates maximally stress the system and may reveal a covert obstruction (Fig. 6.5). The normal pyeloureteral unit can accept these rates without an abnormal pressure rise; ureters having successful surgical correction have provided this perfusion data by acting as their own controls.

Following completion of the study the bladder catheter and renal needle are removed. We have not found it necessary to place the patient on bedrest either in the hospital or at home. We have discontinued, for several years, post-procedural blood pressure and pulse recordings if the examination was uneventful.

Interpretation

Simple subtraction of the bladder pressure from the renal pelvis pressure gives the pressure drop or differential pressure. We have considered differential pressures

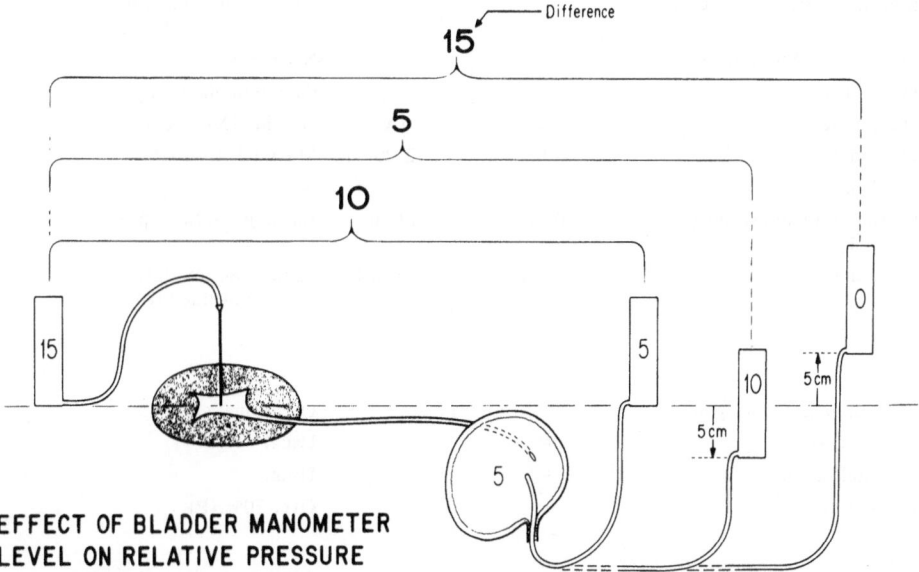

EFFECT OF BLADDER MANOMETER LEVEL ON RELATIVE PRESSURE

Fig. 6.6. Both the renal and bladder pressure recorders (manometer bases) should be level with the tip of the kidney needle. During perfusion, and at a bladder pressure of 5 cmH$_2$O, the differential pressure is 10 cmH$_2$O. Lowering or raising the bladder pressure recorder by 5 cm will result in differential pressures of 5 and 15 cmH$_2$O, respectively. Such extraneous factors must be avoided or inaccurate perfusion pressure values will occur. (Pfister and Newhouse 1979.)

Table 6.3. Contraindications to ureteral perfusion

1)	Bleeding diathesis
2)	Active urinary infection
3)	High-grade or complete obstruction
4)	Vesicoureteral reflux without trapping (ipsilateral)

Table 6.4. Comparative features of percutaneous techniques

Item	Whitaker (W)	Pfister (P)	Comment
Equipment			
Pressure transducer	+	–	Requires manometer calibration
Chart recorder	+	–	Cumbersome
Water manometers	–	+	Simple, quick
Needle/catheter size	18 gT	22g	Catheter sheathed needle (W)
Infusion pump heads	single	dual	Dual cheaper than two singles for bilateral studies
Conduct			
Calculation resistance needle/catheter	+	–	Necessary with small bore unit recordings
Constant pressure monitoring	+	– +	Single 22g needle (P) Double 22g needle (P)
Immediate preceding VCUG	–	+	Excludes intermittent significant reflux (P)
Fluoroscopic monitoring	+	+	Necessary
IV contrast	+	–	Only nondilated (P)
Study time	2X	1X	30 min (1X), average
Flow rates ml/min	2–10	2–20	Maximal stress (P)
Sterile urine	+	+	Necessary
Maximum renal pressure (cmH$_2$O)	50–80	40–50	Intrarenal reflux 30–50
Perfusate	Saline or contrast	Contrast	Saline leak invisible, not recommended (P)
Patient			
NPO	+	+	4 h
General anaesthesia, young	+	–	Occasional (W)
Sedation, young	+	+	Usual
Hospitalisation	+	–	Usual
Outpatient	–	+	Over 70% (P)
Results			
Permanent record	Graph	Written	Equivalent data
Morbidity	+	+	Minimal; pain, haematuria, sepsis
Renal loss	–	–	
Mortality	–	–	

below 12 cmH_2O as normal; 12-14 cmH_2O as equivocal and 15 cmH_2O or greater as evidence of obstruction (Pfister and Newhouse 1979; Whitaker 1973). As indicated previously, free-flowing pressures must also be obtained and pressure recorders (manometers) have to be set at the level of the tip of the renal needle (Fig. 6.6). Perfusion runs must be done with the bladder empty and full; in some cases, obstruction will be evident only when the bladder is distended, although most abnormal differential pressures are apparent with an empty bladder.

Contraindications

Bleeding is the most serious complication of PFS and we consider a blood coagulation disorder a contraindication to the procedure. Table 6.3 lists other situations where PFS are to be avoided.

Conclusions

Physiological information on the ability of the ureter to transport or conduct urine to a reservoir (bladder, loop, intact colon, skin) may be obtained by pressure flow studies. While precise quantification of resistance is possible, the exact values of differential pressure between the kidney and reservoir in normal systems and mild obstruction are still undergoing investigation. Our experience now exceeds 620 percutaneous perfusion pressure flow studies (155 on PUJ problems) and our approach has been to make them simple and safe; as a result, 70% are now performed on an outpatient basis. Additionally, higher flow-rates than those described by Whitaker have been incorporated into the procedure; these and other modifications have been found to be clinically valuable (Table 6.4).

Acknowledgements. The author would like to acknowledge the help and cooperation he has received during this study from the following colleagues: Dr Stephen P. Dretler, Dr Jeffrey H. Newhouse, Dr W. Hardy Hendren, Dr. Isobel C. Yoder and Dr Alex F. Althausen.

References

Koff SA, Thrall JH, Keyes JW Jr (1979) Diuretic radionuclide urography: A noninvasive method for evaluating nephroureteral dilatation. J Urol 122: 451–454

Koff SA, Thrall JH, Keyes JW Jr (1980) Assessment of hydroureteronephrosis in children using diuretic radionuclide urography. J Urol 123: 531–534

O'Reilly PH, Lawson RS, Shields RA, Testa HJ (1979) Idiopathic hydronephrosis—the diuresis renogram: A new non-invasive method of assessing equivocal pyeloureteral junction obstruction. J Urol 121: 153–155

O'Reilly PH, Testa HJ, Lawson RS, Farrar DJ, Edwards EC (1978) Diuresis renography in equivocal urinary tract obstruction. Br J Urol 50: 76–80

Pfister RC (1978) Ureterodynamics. Dialogues in Pediatric Urology 1/10: 3–4

Pfister RC, Newhouse JH (1978) Radiology of ureter. Urology 12: 15–39

Pfister RC, Newhouse JH (1979) Interventional percutaneous pyeloureteral techniques. I. Antegrade pyelography and ureteral perfusion. Radiol Clin North Am 17: 341–350

Pfister RC, Newhouse JH, Yoder IC (1980) Effect of flow rates on ureteral perfusion results. Am J Roentgenol 135: 209

Weiss RM, Schiff M Jr, Lytton B (1976) Reflux and trapping. Radiology 118: 129–131

Whitaker RH (1973) Methods of assessing obstruction in dilated ureters. Br J Urol 45: 15–22

Whitaker RH (1975) Equivocal pelvi-ureteric obstruction. Br J Urol 47: 771–779

Whitaker RH (1976) Investigating wide ureters with ureteral pressure flow studies. J Urol 116: 81–82

Whitaker RH (1978) Clinical assessment of pelvic and ureteral function. Urology 12: 146–150

Whitaker RH (1979a) An evaluation of 170 diagnostic pressure flow studies in the upper urinary tract. J Urol 121: 602–604

Whitaker RH (1979b) Clinical application of upper urinary tract dynamics. Urol Clin North Am 6: 137–141

Whitaker RH (1979c) The Whitaker test. Urol Clin North Am 6: 529–539

Whitfield HN, Britton KE, Fry IK, Hendry WF, Nimmon CC, Travers P, Wickham JEA (1977) The obstructed kidney: Correlation between renal function and urodynamic assessment. Br J Urol 49: 615–619

Yoder IC, Pfister RC (1978) Radiology of colon loop diversion: Anatomical and urodynamic studies of the conduit and ureters in children and adults. Radiology 127: 85–92

7. Experimental Validation of Diagnostic Methods

S.A. Koff

Chapters 4–6 describe two diagnostic tests, namely diuresis renography and perfusion pressure flow studies, which have been used in the evaluation of idiopathic hydronephrosis. While not defining obstruction, both techniques utilise empiric criteria for identifying the obstructed kidney and distinguishing it from one which is dilated but not obstructed. The following experimental studies are presented in an attempt to determine the validity of these techniques, to identify their inaccuracies and to establish their role in the overall management of patients with idiopathic hydronephrosis.

One of the major potential problems with new diagnostic tests is that individual and institutional enthusiasm may generate occult biases which escape detection. Consequently, the results of such tests may become self-serving and appear to perpetuate spuriously high degrees of accuracy. Tests which assess obstruction in hydronephrosis are susceptible to these hazards because whenever a kidney is diagnosed as being obstructed, an operation is generally performed and some form of ureteral or ureteropelvic abnormality may be encountered. While this apparently 'proves' that the test was accurate, one must seriously wonder what would happen to these kidneys if they remained without the benefit of an operation.

Complete scientific validation of diagnostic tests which supposedly distinguish between obstructive and non-obstructive hydronephrosis must ultimately depend on not operating upon kidneys which satisfy the criteria for obstruction and observing their progressive deterioration. While such a planned prospective protocol is obviously unconscionable in humans, it is feasible in experimental animals. The following is an evaluation of several diagnostic methods for assessing obstruction in the dilated urinary tract in a canine model with partial ureteral obstruction.

Materials and Methods

Incomplete ureteral ligation was performed under intravenous sodium pentobarbitol anaesthesia in 12 adult female mongrel dogs weighing 15–25 kg. The ureter was isolated transperitoneally, approximately 2–4 cm from the ureterovesical junction and partially occluded with a 2-0 silk ligature. An 18g needle was placed alongside the ureter during ligation and thereafter removed to ensure that the ligation was incomplete. A constriction, but not a complete occlusion of the ureter, was produced by this technique. In six dogs contralateral nephrectomy was also performed.

The animals were studied pre-operatively and post-operatively at approximately 2-week intervals until either the renal pelvic volume exceeded 100 ml or there was evidence of uraemia. The silk ligature was then surgically removed and thereafter the animals were again studied at periodic intervals.

The progress of hydronephrosis was assessed in all dogs by the following methods:

1) Serum renal function tests (blood urea nitrogen (BUN) and creatinine)
2) Intravenous urography including delayed films
3) Diuresis renography
4) Urodynamic tests
      Resting intrapelvic pressure
      Resting intrapelvic volume
      Perfusion pressure flow studies

All tests except biochemical studies were performed under intravenous sodium pentobarbitol anaesthesia. A 10-day course of parenteral antibiotics (chloramphenicol 50 mg/kg) was used after each operative study session.

The technique of diuresis renography has been previously reported (Koff et al. 1979). Briefly, each dog received intravenously a weight-adjusted dose of 99m-technetium labelled DTPA (0.14 mCi/kg and was studied in the prone position by means of the gamma-scintillation camera. After tracer injection the gamma camera oscilloscope and scintiphotos were monitored to determine when the renal collecting structures (pelvis and calyces) were visualised. Frusemide 0.3 mg/kg was injected intravenously and data collection continued for an additional 15 min. After all data were stored in the nuclear medicine minicomputer (2 frames/min), the results were inspected frame by frame to select those frames of particular interest. The individual regions of interest were the entire kidney (including the pelvis) and the ureter. Background corrected time-activity curves for each kidney and ureter were then generated, and compared with the previously reported normal, dilated but not obstructed, and obstructed patterns (Fig. 7.1).

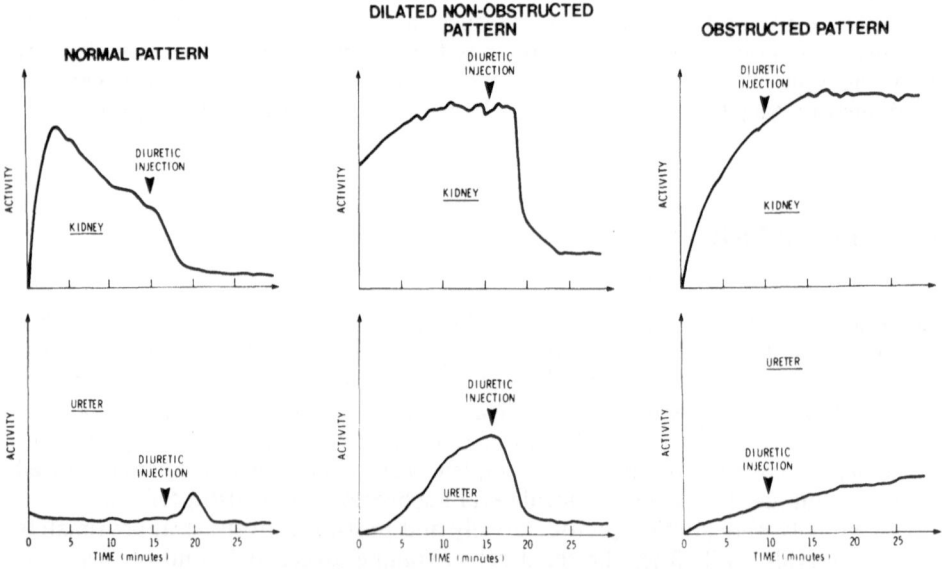

Fig. 7.1. Diuresis renography. Time activity patterns for kidney and ureter illustrating the normal, dilated non-obstructed, and obstructed patterns.

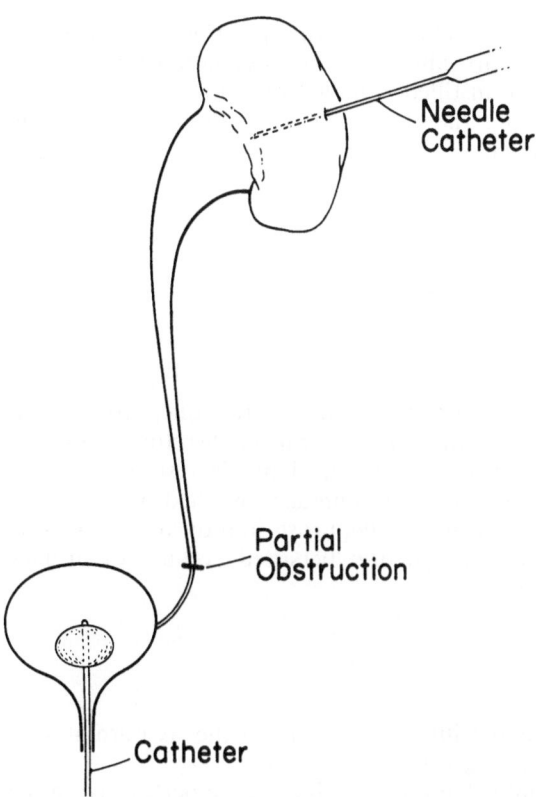

Fig. 7.2. Schematic representation of the experimental design for urodynamic study of the partially obstructed canine kidney.

The kidney was exposed but not mobilised via an upper midline or flank incision for each set of urodynamic studies. A balloon-type urethral catheter was inserted into the bladder and connected to a water manometer which recorded intravesical pressure.

Resting intrapelvic pressure was measured in a state of antidiuresis in an inertia-free system which employed a 16g silastic needle catheter (Abbocath) connected to a commercial recording carbon dioxide cystometer with a continuous flow rate of 5 ml/min. With the gas flowing, the needle catheter was thrust into the renal pelvis through the renal parenchyma and the intrapelvic pressure was recorded. In some cases with high intrapelvic pressure, a small amount of urine would backfill the catheter lumen following intrapelvic placement. In these cases, the value for resting intrapelvic pressure was the pressure recorded after the urine (<1 cm^3) had been replaced into the pelvis (Fig. 7.2).

After measurement of intrapelvic pressure, all urine contained within the kidney, renal pelvis and ureter was aspirated through the needle catheter and the volume was recorded as the pelviureteric volume. Volume was also measured in six non-obstructed nephroureteral systems at the time of nephrectomy.

Perfusion pressure flow studies were performed and repeated according to the methods described by Whitaker (1973) by perfusing saline through the needle catheter at 10 ml/min using a Harvard pump. The infusion pressure was monitored with an in-line water manometer and, after correcting for intravesical pressure and the measured internal resistance of the system, the actual perfusion pressure was obtained and recorded. In all instances, the saline infusion was continued for several minutes after the volume of perfusate instilled equalled the previously measured pelviureteric volume. After completing the perfusion pressure flow study, the pelviureteric volume was again measured.

Results

General

Incomplete ureteral ligation produced a progressive hydroureteronephrosis in all experimental animals. In two dogs with contralateral nephrectomy, rapidly progressive uraemia and death occurred prior to urodynamic testing. Surgical removal of ureteric sutures was performed in ten animals; one died before upper tract urodynamics could be assessed. Hydroureteronephrosis improved in all but one dog after suture removal. In this case obstruction persisted because of urinary extravasation at the site of the suture.

Renal Pelviureteric Volume

The volume of urine contained in the pelviureteric systems of the six normal non-dilated nephrectomised urinary tracts ranged from 3 to 5 cm^3.

Thirty-seven measurements of renal pelviureteric volume were performed in ten animals during the development of hydroureteronephrosis and are recorded in Fig. 7.3. A near-linear progressive increase in measured volume occurred in all dogs. At the time of suture removal the volumes ranged from 81 to 512 cm^3.

Following successful suture removal in nine survivors, seven pelviureteric systems returned to a resting volume of 10 cm^3 or less, while two systems remained dilated. In one of the persistently dilated systems (75 cm^3) obstruction from urinary extravasation was demonstrated; in the other dilated system (37 cm^3) no obstruction was evident.

Renal Function Studies

In six dogs with partial ureteral ligation and contralateral nephrectomy, 112 separate renal function studies were performed. Control pre-operative values for serum creatinine ranged from 0.6 to 1.2 mg/dl (mean 1.0) and blood urea nitrogen ranged from 10 to 21 mg/dl (mean 15).

Figure 7.4 illustrates the patterns of serum creatinine elevation in dogs with one kidney during the development of hydroureteronephrosis. Except for one dog with a rapid impairment in renal function, the remaining animals displayed a plateau of slightly elevated creatinine values for a number of weeks following ligation. Thereafter, rapidly increasing serum creatinine values occurred abruptly in all but one animal. The changes in blood urea nitrogen paralleled those of serum creatinine. An insufficient number of renal function analyses were performed following suture removal.

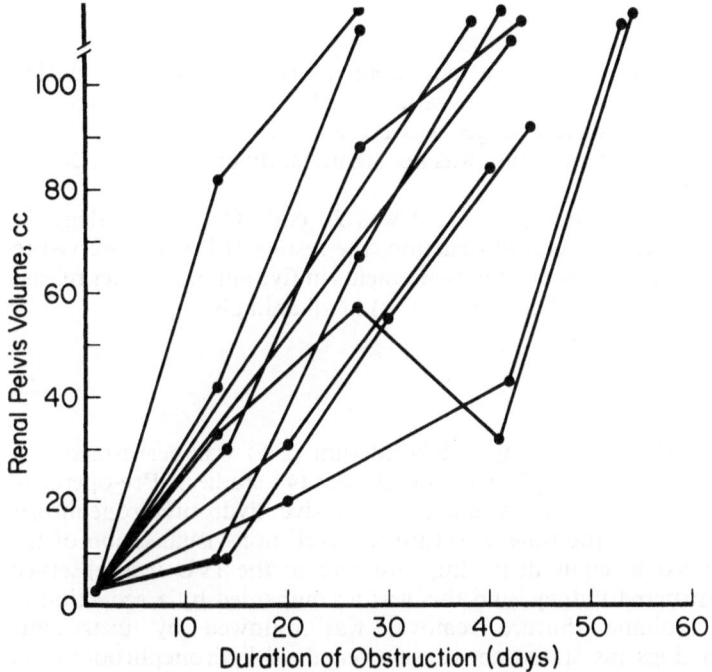

Fig. 7.3. Pelviureteric volume changes following incomplete ureteral ligation.

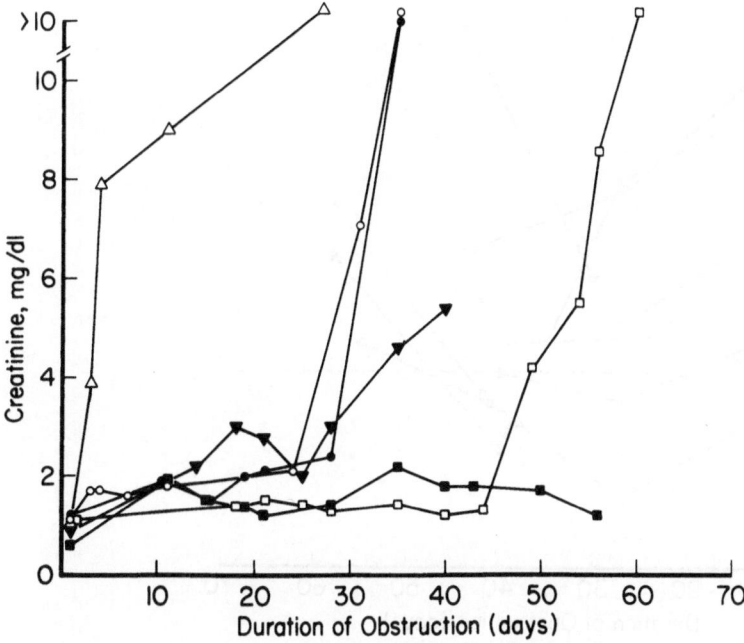

Fig. 7.4. Effect of partial ureteral ligation and contralateral nephrectomy on serum creatinine.

Intrapelvic Pressure

Thirty-seven resting intrapelvic pressure measurements (IPP) were made during progressive hydroureteronephrosis. The alterations in IPP were individualised and variable, and no trend in pressure changes was evident (Fig. 7.5). Mean pressure at 2, 4 and 6 weeks following obstruction was not significantly different (31, 26 and 27 cmH_2O respectively).

The upper limit of normal for resting IPP was 20 cmH_2O (15.4 mmHg). In hydronephrotic systems with ureteral obstruction, the resting IPP was observed to be within the normal range in eight of 25 measurements in five animals. After release of obstruction IPP was normal (15 cmH_2O or less) in all animals.

Intravenous Urography

Intravenous urography (IVU) including a delayed film (2 h) was performed pre-operatively and at intervals post-operatively in all dogs (46 studies). Pre-operative examinations were normal in each animal. Progressive hydroureteronephrosis developed in all dogs, and at the time of suture removal, non-visualisation of the affected kidney occurred in eight dogs. Improvement in the IVU was observed transiently in one obstructed kidney, and this was accompanied by a reduction in resting pelviureteric volume. Suture removal was followed by urographic improvement in eight dogs (as stated above, one remained hydronephrotic) (Fig. 7.6).

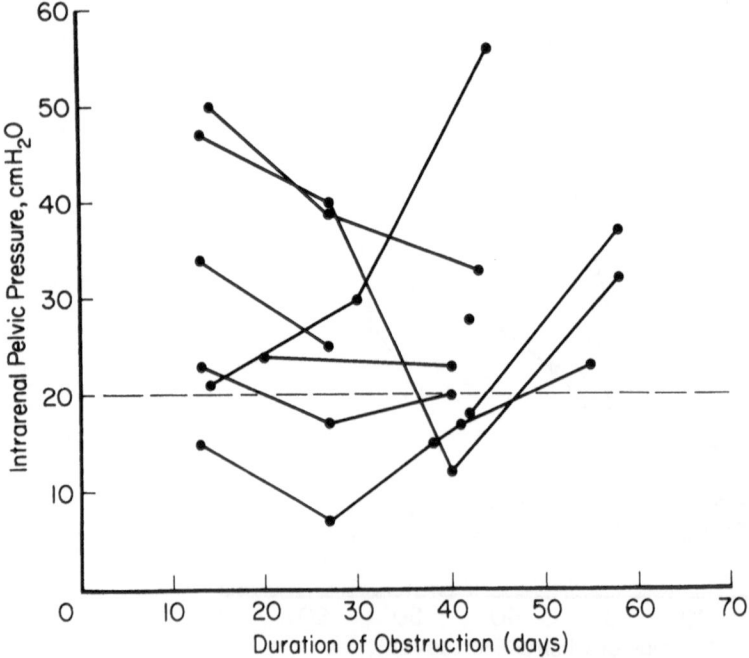

Fig. 7.5. Measurements of intrapelvic pressure after partial ureteral ligation.

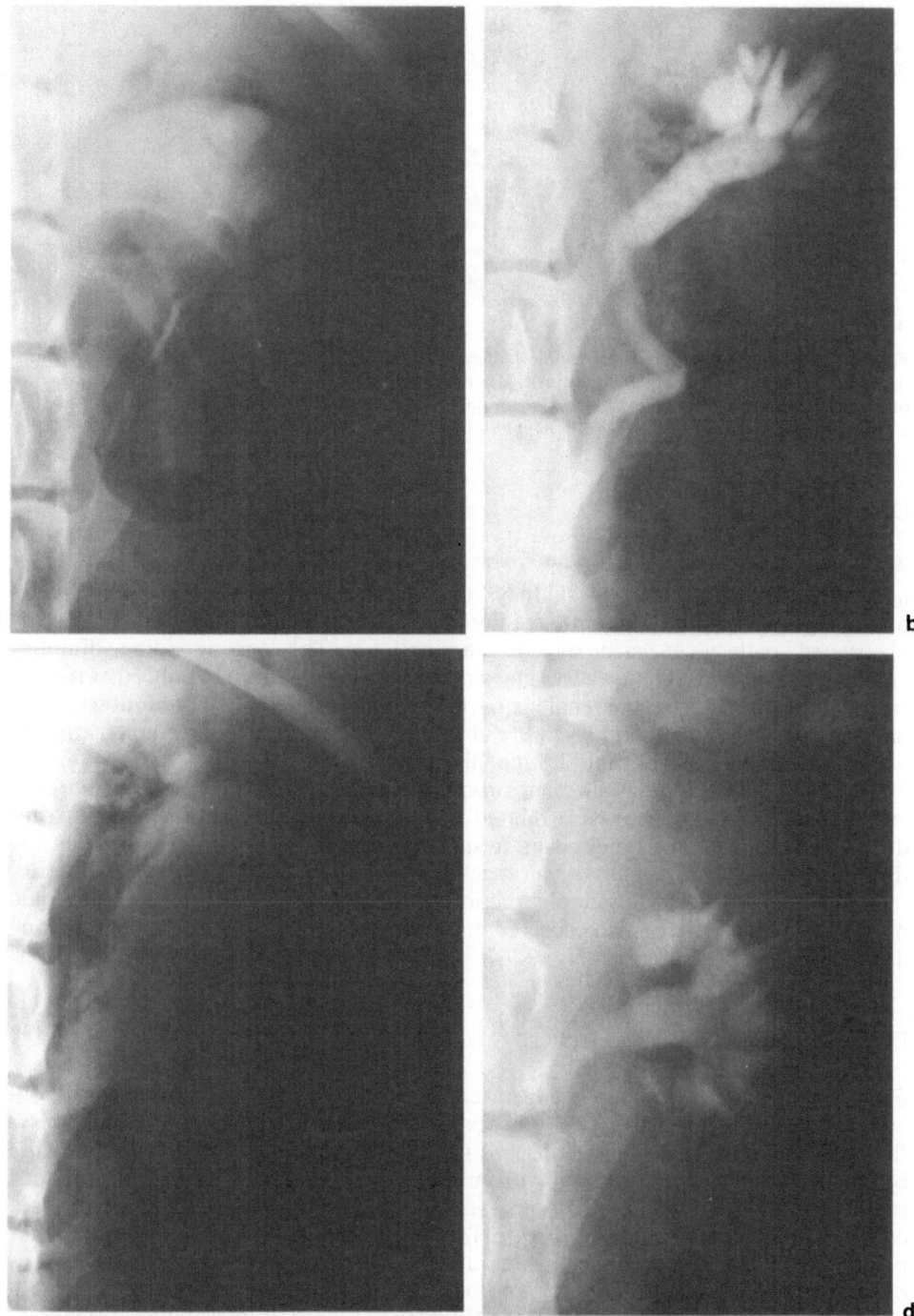

Fig. 7.6. Serial intravenous pyelograms in a canine kidney subjected to ureteral ligation and then suture removal pre-operatively (**a**); 2 weeks after partial ureteral ligation (**b**); 1 month later — non-visualising mass (**c**); and 2 weeks after suture removal (**d**). Note similar degrees of hydroureteronephrosis before **b** and after suture removal (**d**).

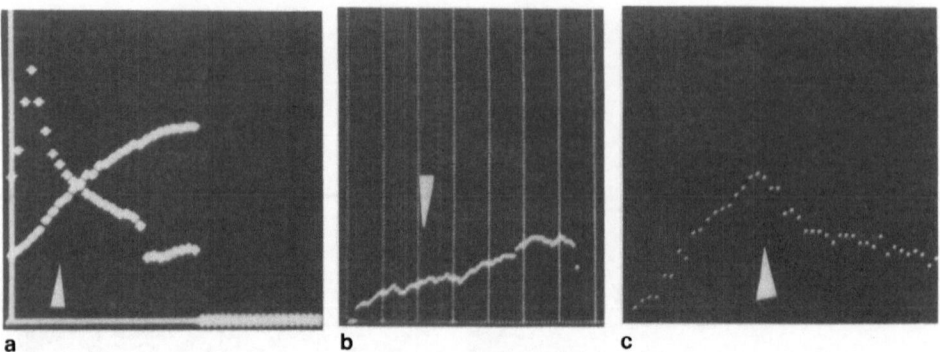

Fig. 7.7. Diuresis renography of a canine kidney after partial ureteral obstruction (*arrows* indicate timing of diuretic injection): **a** Two weeks after ligation the obstructed kidney demonstrates the obstructed pattern, contralateral kidney is normal. **b** One month later obstructed pattern persists. **c** Two weeks after suture removal the dilated, non-obstructed pattern is registered.

Diuresis Renography

A total of 109 diuresis renograms were performed, including 31 examinations of normal non-obstructed canine kidneys and ureters (Fig. 7.1). In ten dogs with obstructed ureters, the diuretic radionuclide *ureteral* study demonstrated an obstructed pattern in each of 24 examinations. The corresponding diuretic radionuclide *renal* study, however, showed an obstructed pattern in only 20 of the 24 studies. In four instances the renal histogram registered a dilated but non-obstructed pattern. All four of these kidneys were visibly hydronephrotic and serum creatinine values ranged between 1.4 and 2.8 mg/dl (mean 2.1 mg/dl).

Following suture removal in nine surviving animals, *renal and ureteral* diuresis renography ultimately showed a dilated but non-obstructed pattern in six of the dogs. The average time required after suture removal for diuresis renography to display washout was 5 weeks with a range of 2–12 weeks. Renal and ureteral diuresis renography in two dogs without obstruction continued to demonstrate an obstructed pattern; a similar pattern also occurred in a third animal with persisting obstruction due to urinary extravasation (Fig. 7.7).

Perfusion Pressure Flow Studies

Forty perfusion pressure flow studies were performed and a perfusion pressure of >22 cmH$_2$O was used to define an obstructed system (Fig. 7.8). Pressures less than 15 cmH$_2$O were considered normal; values of 15–22 cmH$_2$O were considered to be equivocal. During progressive hydroureteronephrosis, pressure in the obstructed range occured in 20 studies in six dogs, while pressures in the equivocal range (15–22 cmH$_2$O) were noted in six studies in four dogs. Following suture removal the perfusion pressures were in the normal range in 12 studies in seven dogs, and in the obstructed range in two studies in two dogs.

After completing perfusion pressure flow studies in three dogs whose pressures equilibrated in the non-obstructed range, the entire pelviureteric system was aspirated and the volume measured. The recovered volumes represented 84%–95% of the volumes of perfusate instilled during the perfusion.

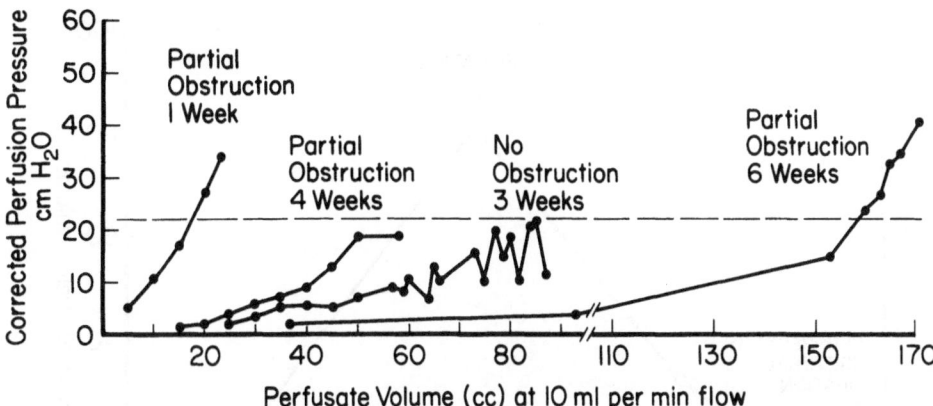

Fig. 7.8. Perfusion pressure flow studies performed sequentially in a canine kidney subjected to partial ureteral ligation and then suture removal. Potential for error exists if the large, dilated system is not filled to physiologic capacity; equilibration of pressures in the normal range may simulate no obstruction.

Discussion

The aims of this study were first to produce a canine model with partial ureteral obstruction and progressive hydroureteronephrosis, and then to examine the accuracy and to identify the pitfalls of the clinical diagnostic methods currently used to assess obstruction in the upper urinary tract. Success was achieved in producing an incomplete obstruction by using a partially occluding ligature, but the degree of obstruction was variable; upper tract dilatation proceeded at different rates and three dogs died before all testing was complete. Progression of hydro-ureteronephrosis, however, occurred in all kidneys with partially ligated ureters and was documented by serial measurements of enlarging pelviureteric volumes. That the obstruction was incomplete was confirmed by recovering perfusate from the urinary bladder following pressure flow studies. Additionally, the rate at which the pelviureteric systems expanded served as a time frame upon which to evaluate the other diagnostic tests.

Although serum renal function studies are often used clinically to follow patients with hydroureteronephrosis, they were not reliable in assessing the progress of canine urinary tract obstruction. Sequential measurements in single kidney animals with partial ureteral occlusion clearly indicated that mild elevations of serum creatinine (1.4–2.2 mg/dl) and BUN could be maintained while the upper tract progressively dilated (Figs. 7.4 and 7.9). Consequently, elevations of serum creatinine in this range were of no value in either following hydronephrosis to determine whether progressive changes were occurring, or predicting whether or when severe renal insufficiency would ensue. Likewise, persistence of normal or minimally elevated serum creatinine levels for a period of weeks was no insurance that renal function would not abruptly worsen.

Canine intravenous urograms accurately registered progression of hydro-ureteronephrosis, but similar degrees of dilatation were regularly observed in the same renal unit before and after suture removal. Therefore, each intravenous urographic study was of no value in predicting whether hydroureteronephrosis was improving. However, when the intravenous urograms in each animal were viewed as

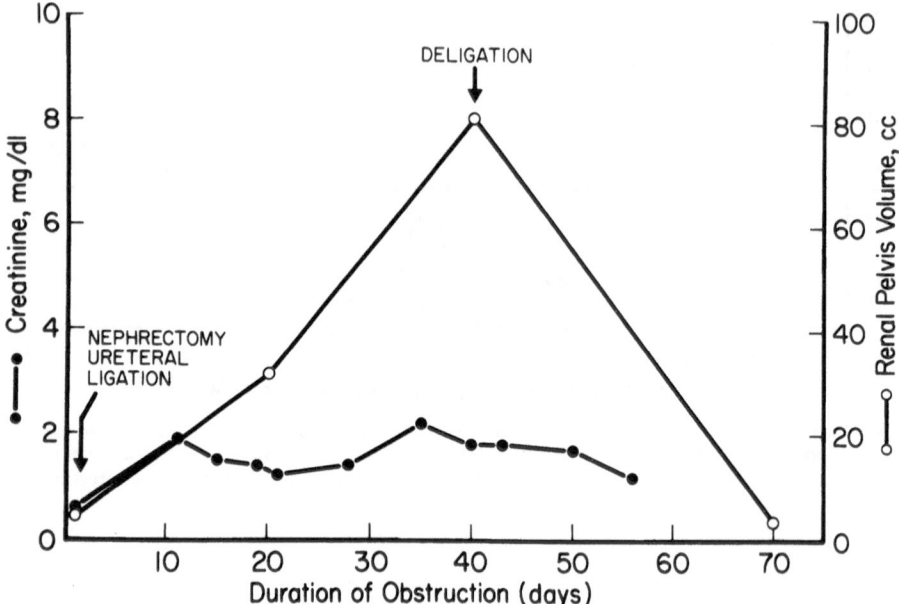

Fig. 7.9. Serum creatinine and pelviureteric volume measurements in a one-kidney dog, subjected to partial ureteral ligation and then suture removal (deligation), indicate that mild elevations of serum creatinine can be maintained while the upper tract progressively dilates.

a collective series, they were consistently effective in all dogs in recording pelviureteric volume changes, and were accurate in determining whether hydroureteronephrosis was progressing or improving. An exception to this occurred when poor renal function and urographic non-visualisation made comparisons between kidneys impossible.

Although elevated intrapelvic pressure is considered to be pathogenetic in producing hydronephrotic renal damage, measurements of pressure in chronic hydronephrosis are often normal (Hinman 1970; Backlund et al. 1965; Djurhuus and Stage 1976a; Schweitzer 1973). The reported time course of intrapelvic pressure changes following total canine ureteral occlusion shows a return from elevated to normal pressures within days or weeks (Vaughan et al. 1970); this reflects a severe impairment in renal function with a resulting inability to generate high hydrostatic pressures (Rose and Gillenwater 1978). Previous reports of intrapelvic pressure measurements in animals with partial ureteral obstruction have described a similar trend toward normal pressures with duration of obstruction (Schweitzer 1973; Djurhuus et al. 1976b; Weaver 1968; Boyarsky and Martinez 1964). This appears paradoxical because renal function is usually less severely affected during experimental partial obstruction, and elevated intrapelvic pressures should be registered at least intermittently. An alternative explanation in such cases is that sustained normal intrapelvic pressure during partial occlusion reflects an insufficient degree of obstruction to produce a progressive impairment in renal function. This is supported by noting that although an initial deterioration in renal function and/or hydronephrosis occurred in many of the reported animals with partial obstruction, true progression of these abnormalities rarely was documented (Schweitzer 1973; Djurhuus et al. 1976b; Boyarsky and Martinez 1964; Olesen and Madsen 1968).

In contrast with these previous reports, the present work has shown that animals with documented progressive hydroureteronephrosis demonstrate no tendency for normalisation of intrapelvic pressures, which fluctuate widely as a function of time. This seemingly erratic intrapelvic pressure response to partial ureteral obstruction may reflect periodic overdistension of the renal pelvis which produces elevated pressures that are important in the pathogenesis of hydronephrotic renal damage. This repetitive process of overdistension of the renal pelvis with measurably increased pressures and impaired renal function (followed by gradual emptying, and then refilling and improvement in renal function) is probably the common mechanism by which all incompletely obstructed nephroureteral systems undergo progressive and sizeable hydronephrotic dilatation while still preserving renal function (Hinman 1970; Koff et al. 1980). Eventually if an equilibrium state is not reached, the additive effects of intermittent raised intrapelvic pressures would cause renal function to deteriorate, at times abruptly, as it did in our experimental animals.

Intrapelvic pressure was normal at some time during the progression of hydroureteronephrosis in 50% of the experimental animals. Measurement of pressure, therefore, was of limited value in predicting whether or not urinary tract dilatation was progressive.

Canine perfusion pressure flow studies, performed according to Whitaker's technique and criteria (Whitaker 1973), were able to identify obstruction in only six of ten dogs in 20 of 26 studies. Overlap in perfusion pressures between normal and partially obstructed ureters has been previously reported in experimental animals (Koff 1978). After relief of obstruction, however, the test was more successful in recognising a non-obstructed system. In attempting to identify a cause for these false-negative results, we observed that large volumes of perfusate were recovered by aspiration from the obstructed pelviureteric systems of those dogs whose perfusion pressures equilibrated in the non-obstructed range (84%–95% of the instilled perfusate). This finding indicates that while there was filling of the renal pelvis and ureter, very little fluid passed across the site of obstruction, and this is at variance with the original premise that 'the pressure which is recorded is that pressure necessary to drive the fluid through the system at a fixed flow rate' (Whitaker 1973). Examination of pressure flow studies in each animal at periodic intervals supported the fact that pelviureteric filling and volume expansion may occur at normal pressures without propulsion of significant amounts of fluid across the ureteral obstruction; the pressures recorded were filling pressures rather than true pressure flow values. This may simulate equilibration of pressures in the normal or non-obstructed range and result in a falsely negative test interpretation (Fig. 7.8). In order to remedy this potential problem, especially in large-volume dilated systems, perfusion must be continued for a sufficiently long period of time to fill the pelvis and ureter to their physiological capacity before normal pressures are accepted as validly indicating absence of obstruction.

Previous reports on the use of diuresis renography have suggested that the ureteral histogram is more accurate than is the renal histogram in assessing ureteral (rather than PUJ) obstruction (Koff et al. 1979, 1980). This was confirmed in our study: during obstruction all ureteral histograms demonstrated obstruction, whereas four of 24 renal histograms showed no obstruction. For maximum accuracy, therefore, regions of interest must be selected from the area of dilatation nearest and proximal to the site of obstruction, in this case the distal ureter, and in idiopathic hydronephrosis, the renal pelvis.

Soon after release of obstruction the diuresis renogram was temporarily inaccurate and often did not demonstrate washout of tracer until renal function had recovered to a level where frusemide injection would produce a diuresis (2–12 weeks after suture removal). In two animals, the renal and ureteral histograms continued to demonstrate an obstructed pattern in the absence of organic obstruction, but in both instances a severe renal functional impairment persisted.

In attempting to extrapolate from these canine studies to clinical hydronephrosis, one must carefully consider that renal pathologic changes develop and resolve much more rapidly in the dog than in the human. As a result, alterations that occur abruptly in the dog may progress at a slower rate in the human kidney, while those changing slowly in the canine may be altered imperceptibly or not at all in man. Any of the diagnostic studies, therefore, which depend on serial changes such as serum renal function study and intrapelvic pressure and volume may be less accurate in humans because the changes occur more slowly; therefore the results of the present studies must be extrapolated with caution.

The three most accurate methods for assessing canine ureteral obstruction were serial intravenous pyelography, diuresis renography and perfusion pressure flow studies. In human investigations, the intravenous pyelogram is consistently less helpful because often this is only a single examination, and the risk of waiting for evidence of progressive destruction is usually not acceptable, especially in children. The latter two methods, however, have been shown to be particularly effective in investigating hydronephrosis. In examining their tendencies for false-positive or false-negative results, we find that the diuresis renogram and the perfusion pressure flow examination are complementary in clinical practice: when impaired renal function prevents a diuresis and therefore tracer washout the perfusion study is unaffected. When perfusion pressures appear normal in large capacity obstructed systems, choice of a region of interest near the obstruction will often make the radionuclide study more accurate.

References

Backlund L, Grotte G, Reuterskiold A (1965) Functional stenosis as a cause of pelviureteric junction obstruction and hydronephrosis. Arch Dis Child 40: 203

Boyarsky S, Martinez J (1964) Pathophysiology of the ureter: Partial ligation of the ureter in dogs. Invest Urol 2: 173

Djurhuus JC, Stage P (1976) Percutaneous intrapelvic pressure registration in hydronephrosis during diuresis. Acta Chir Scand 472: 43

Djurhuus JC, Nerstrom B, Gyrd-Hansen N, Rask Anderson H (1976) Experimental hydronephrosis. Acta Chir Scand 472: 17

Hinman F Jr (1970) The pathophysiology of urinary obstruction. In: Campbell MF, Harrison JH (ed) Urology. Saunders, Philadelphia, pp 313–348

Koff SA (1978) Experimental assessment of graded ureteral obstruction utilizing liquid and gaseous perfusion techniques. Invest Urol 16: 229

Koff SA, Thrall JH, Keyes JW Jr (1979) Diuretic radionuclide urography: A non-invasive method of evaluating nephroureteral dilation. J Urol 122: 451

Koff SA, Thrall JH, Keyes JW Jr (1980) Assessment of hydroureteronephrosis in children utilizing diuretic radionuclide urography. J Urol 123: 531

Olesen S, Madsen PO (1968) Function during partial obstruction following contralateral nephrectomy in the dog. J Urol 99: 692

Rose JG, Gillenwater JY (1978) Effects of obstruction on ureteral function. Urology 12: 139

Schweitzer FAW (1973) Intrapelvic pressure and renal function studies in experimental chronic partial ureteric obstruction. Br J Urol 45: 2

Vaughan ED Jr, Sorensen EJ, Gillenwater JY (1970) The renal haemodynamic response to chronic
    unilateral complete ureteral occlusion. Invest Urol 8: 78
Weaver RG (1968) Reabsorptive patterns and pressures in hydronephrosis with clinical application. J
    Urol 100: 112
Whitaker RH (1973) Methods of assessing obstruction in dilated ureters. Br J Urol 45: 15

8. Idiopathic Hydronephrosis in Children

J.H. Johnston

At operation for pelvic hydronephrosis in children, the most common findings are pelviureteric angulations of various types. These are unquestionably themselves obstructive, but whether they are the primary lesion or secondary developments has long been the subject of argument. Several morphological anomalies have been described and a variety of pathological concepts have been preferred.

Morphological Anomalies

High Insertion Ureter

The ureter originates high on the pelvis instead of at its most dependent part. Under diuresis the pelvis distends, the ureteric orifice moves higher and a valvular type of obstruction results. With time, the formation of pelviureteric adhesions may maintain the deformity and its obstructive effect.

Aberrant Vessels

The inferior branch of the anterior division of the renal artery crosses in front of the ureter just below the pelviureteric junction on its way to the renal hilum. The artery, generally accompanied by small veins, angulates the ureter on the pelvis. Johnston et al. (1977) found aberrant vessels to be present in 59 (24%) of 238 cases of hydronephrosis in children.

Distensible Pelvis

Whitaker (1975) proposed that hydronephrosis could result from an inherently over-distensible pelvis. Under diuresis, the pelvis dilates so that its walls are unable to co-apt during peristalsis and urine cannot be propelled into the ureter.

Ureteric Stenosis: Dyskinesia

A true stricture at the pelviureteric junction is a rare finding in childhood hydronephrosis but often the upper 1 cm or more of the ureter appears relatively narrow and thin-walled. This may be an isolated finding or, more often, it is associated with a pelviureteric angulation. Various authors have studied the segment of ureter histologically but their findings and interpretations have differed.

Murnaghan (1958) found a preponderance of longitudinally arranged muscle fibres which could prevent propulsion of urine. Foote et al. (1970) noted either an entire absence of muscle or the presence of small, abnormal fibres which would interrupt the peristaltic wave. Notley (1971), using the electron microscope, recorded an excess of intermuscular collagen which could prevent normal ureteric distension and so interfere with pelvic emptying. Generalised connective tissue infiltration in hydronephrosis has been described in detail in Chap. 1.

Fetal Folds

During fetal life the upper end of the ureter usually shows intraluminal invaginations of the musculature. These commonly persist post-natally but ordinarily they are not obstructive and they disappear with the growth of the child. On occasions, however, over-developed folds may be a cause of pelviureteric obstruction. Characteristically in such cases the pelvis retains its conical shape and dependent exit and is less dilated than the calyces.

Ureteric Polyp

A pedunculated polyp composed of fronds of connective tissue covered by transitional epthelium is a rare cause of hydronephrosis in children. The lesion may be visible as an irregular filling defect on urography or may first be discovered only at operation. The polyp is benign so that local excision of the involved segment of ureter, followed by pyeloureterostomy, is all that is needed. A benign transitional cell papilloma of the ureter is an even rarer cause of childhood hydronephrosis than is a polyp; the condition has been recorded by Johnston et al. (1977) and by Mirandi and De Assia (1975).

The Renal Parenchyma

The effect of urinary obstruction on the renal parenchyma depends upon the degree and duration of the obstruction and, in cases in which the obstruction began prenatally, upon the level of maturity of the developing kidney at its time of onset. Much of our knowledge of the mechanisms by which the kidney structure is affected by obstruction has been derived from experimental observations. Matz et al. (1969), working with the pig, noted that loss of renal tissue begins by a pressure effect on and within the renal papillae. Rupture of the ducts of Bellini and of the collecting tubules leads to progressive loss of pyramidal substance. Secondary cortical changes consist of atrophy of the related tubules. Renal blood flow is well maintained at first but is later diminished so that further atrophy and fibrosis follow. Degenerative changes in the interlobular and arcuate arteries were noted in hydronephrotic kidneys in children by Winterburn and France (1972). Renal dysplasia, indicated by the existence of primitive tubules, foci of cartilage and, often, cystic change is a common result of obstructive uropathy dating from prenatal life. It may involve localised areas within a functioning kidney or may replace the entire parenchyma, producing a functionless organ.

The Opposite Kidney: Other Congenital Anomalies

Pelvic hydronephrosis presenting during childhood, and particularly during infancy, is frequently bilateral. In children under 6 months of age, both kidneys were affected in 10 of 33 cases of hydronephrosis in the series of Williams and Karlaftis (1966). With unilateral hydronephrosis, the opposite kidney is often congenitally absent or is the site of cystic dysplasia with non-function. Johnston et al. (1977) reported hydronephrosis of a solitary functioning kidney in 9 of 219 cases.

Pelvic hydronephrosis, and other developmental abnormalities in the urinary tract, are frequent coincidental findings in children with such congenital lesions as cardiac anomalies, imperforate anus and spina bifida. Pyelography is needed routinely in affected infants.

Secondary Pelviureteric Obstruction

Pelviureteric junction obstruction and minor degrees of vesicoureteric reflux can occur coincidentally but gross reflux which severely distends the upper urinary tract can produce pelviureteric angulation and subsequent delay in pelvic emptying. Ordinarily, the angulation is transient, so that there is no obstruction to urinary flow at physiological rates. However, in some instances the angulation becomes fixed by

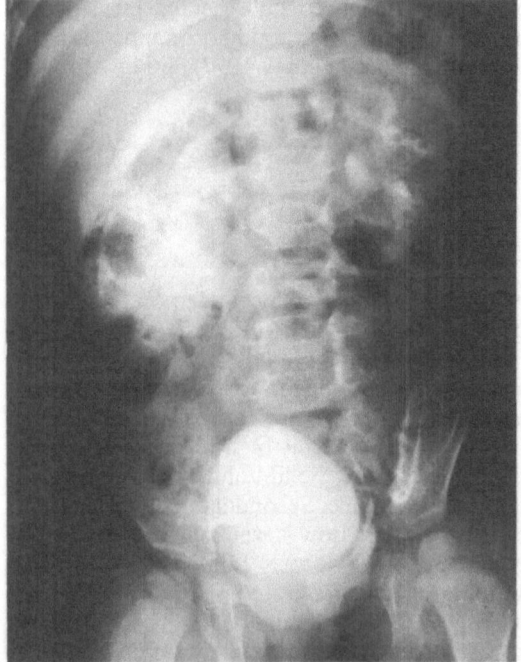
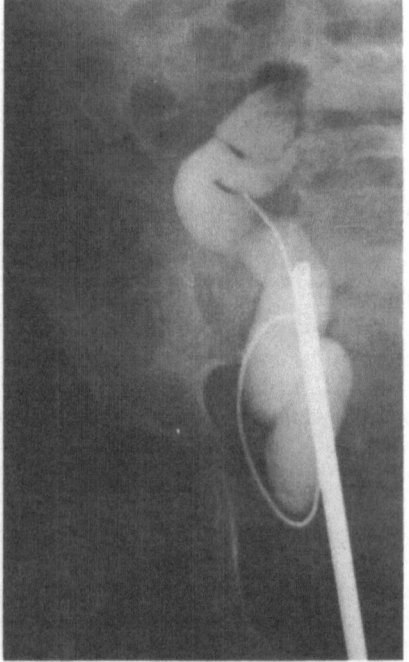

a   b

Fig. 8.1. PUJ obstruction occurring secondary to obstructed megaureter. **a** IVP shows markedly dilated right renal pelvis. **b** Retrograde ureterogram demonstrates dilated, tortuous ureter. Treatment by ureteric remodelling and vesical reimplantation and by pyeloureteroplasty.

adhesions, causing a persistent pelviureteric obstruction necessitating pyeloureteroplasty in addition to operative cure of the reflux. Similar secondary obstructions at the pelviureteric junction may be encountered with megaureters caused by lower ureteric dyskinesia or with dilated ureters associated with an infravesical obstruction (Fig. 8.1).

Complications

Trauma

A large hydronephrotic kidney is more susceptible to trauma and to rupture than a normal one and many hydronephroses in children present for the first time with haematuria following a closed injury. It follows that all kidney injuries in children, even if apparently mild, warrant intravenous urography.

Infection

Bacteraemia may be present in voided specimens, and/or positive urine cultures may be obtained from the urine in a hydronephrotic renal pelvis. However, severe infection leading to a destructive pyonephrosis is a very rare complication.

Calculi

Renal stones developing secondary to hydronephrosis in children are generally composed of calcium phosphate and usually they are small and multiple (Fig. 8.2).

Hypertension

Arterial hypertension is an unusual complication of hydronephrosis during childhood. It is encountered mainly when a solitary kidney is affected. Increased renin secretion occurs chiefly in the early stages of pelviureteric junction obstruction and in chronic cases sodium retention is the responsible factor. In the exceptional case where the contralateral kidney is anatomically normal, it has been considered that there is some defect in its ability to excrete sodium (Vaughan et al. 1974). As a rule the blood pressure returns to normal following pyeloureteroplasty.

Clinical Features

During childhood, pelvic hydronephrosis is found more often in boys than in girls and, when unilateral, the disease is commoner on the left side than on the right. In the series of Johnston et al. (1977) there were 154 boys and 65 girls and the left: right ratio was 139:61.

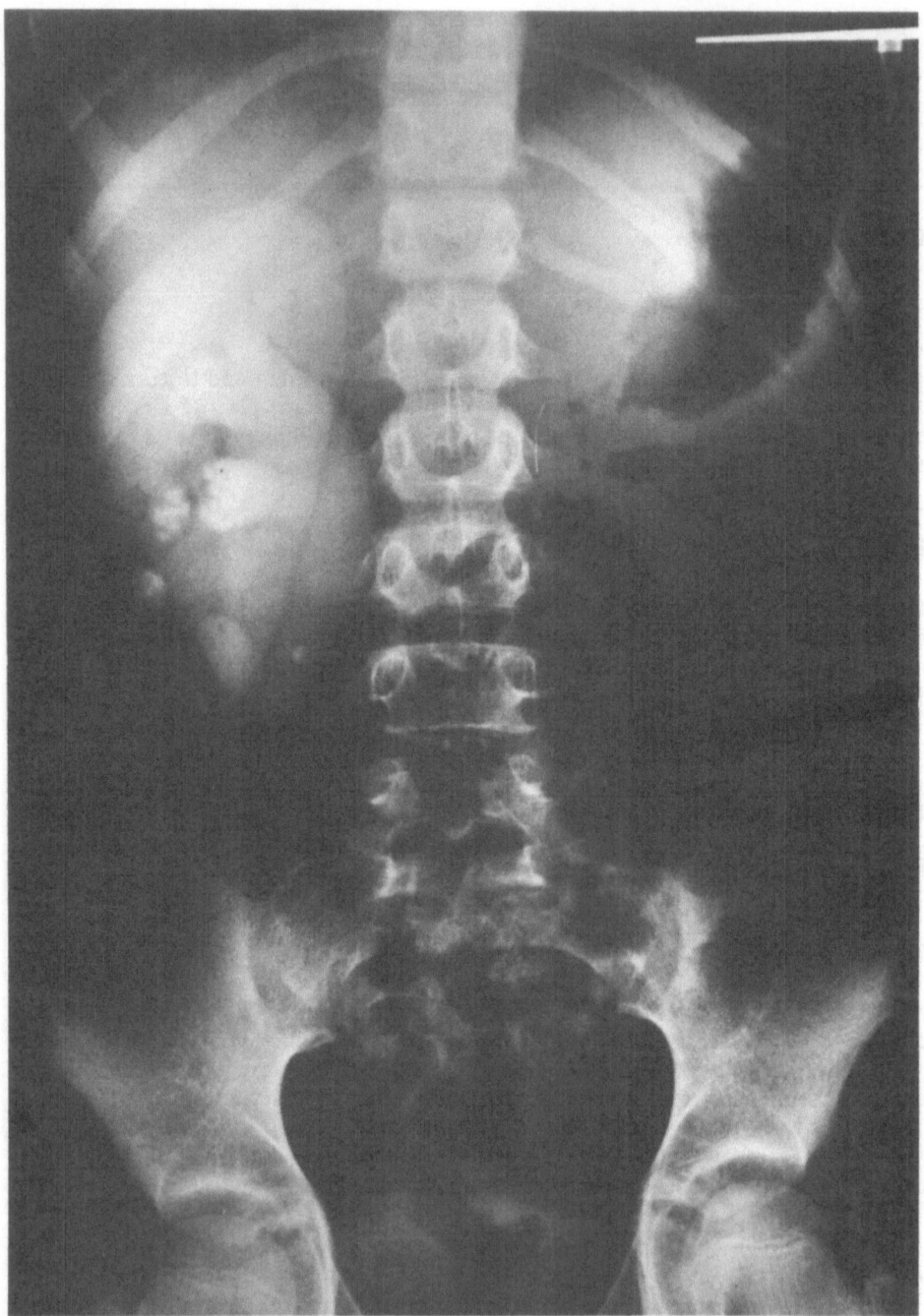

Fig. 8.2. Right hydronephrosis due to PUJ obstruction complicated by the development of multiple small calculi. IVP in an 8-year-old girl. The left kidney showed cystic dysplasia with high ureteric atresia.

In infants, the condition commonly presents as a palpable, or even visible, abdominal mass, often found on routine examination of the newborn. With bilateral disease, or when a solitary kidney is affected, azotaemia and acidaemia may be apparent clinically or on biochemical assessment. Prenatal diagnosis of hydronephrosis is becoming common with the use of ultrasonography during pregnancy.

After infancy, pain, often accompanied by vomiting, is the usual presenting feature. The toddler may refer his discomfort to the umbilical region but the older child complains of pain in the flank. Symptoms of dysuria and fever, suggestive of urinary infection, are common but documented infection is found less frequently; bacteraemia was noted in only 39 of the 219 cases reported by Johnston et al. (1977). Haematuria may occur even in the absence of trauma or calculi. Rarely, hypertension is the presenting feature, either because of its effects or because of its detection on routine clinical examination.

In some instances hydronephrosis is asymptomatic and is found on pyelography performed for disturbances of micturition or in the pyelogram obtained during angiography in children with cardiac anomalies. Genetic factors are involved in the causation of hydronephrosis (Cohen et al. 1978) and, when a strong family history exists, pyelography in an asymptomatic child is fully justified.

Treatment

In adults, it has been stated that pelvic hydronephrosis is often a stable state, without continuing deterioration in renal function (Bratt et al. 1977), and that operation is required only if symptoms exist. In the child, the lesion is more likely to be progressive because of increasing urinary outputs with growth and in my view operative intervention is always indicated even if the patient is asymptomatic.

The operative procedure needed depends on the degree of damage which has already occurred in the kidney and on the prospects for useful recovery of function. When there is no concentration of the contrast on intravenous urography, pre-operative decision on the latter point can be difficult. Most of the methods described for determining function in the individual kidney measure function when obstruction is still present and they are not therefore necessarily of prognostic help. If doubt as to the usefulness of the kidney exists, a brief period of nephrostomy drainage is often valuable in that it allows accurate measurement of the volume and the quality of the urine produced. The size of the hydronephrotic kidney is of little prognostic significance. Particularly in infants, a very large abdominal mass often proves to be produced by a hugely distended pelvis, with a relatively undilated kidney perched on its circumference.

Nephrectomy

Nephrectomy is indicated when the renal parenchyma is irreparably damaged and the kidney is incapable of recovering useful function. As discussed above, pre-operative determination of renal potential can be difficult and the decision as to whether or not nephrectomy is indicated must often be made at operation. Severe cystic dysplasia is a clear indication for nephrectomy, as is the existence of a mere

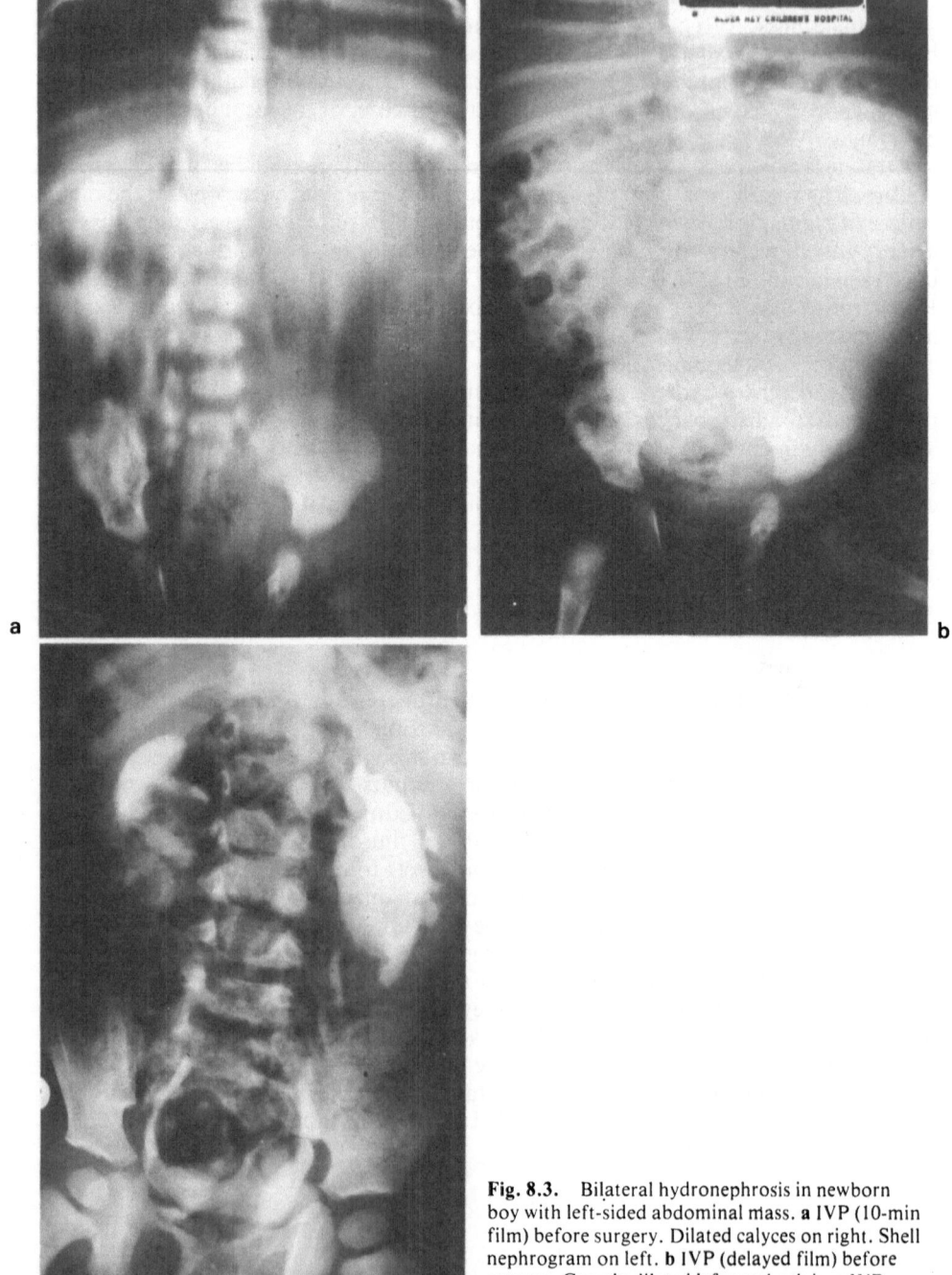

Fig. 8.3. Bilateral hydronephrosis in newborn boy with left-sided abdominal mass. **a** IVP (10-min film) before surgery. Dilated calyces on right. Shell nephrogram on left. **b** IVP (delayed film) before surgery. Grossly dilated left renal pelvis. **c** IVP 2 years after bilateral pyeloureteroplasty showing improved appearances bilaterally.

shell of parenchyma, but otherwise, an assessment should be made, after the pelvis has been emptied, of the total volume of kidney tissue present rather than its thickness alone.

Pyeloureteroplasty

The elimination of angulation at the pelviureteric junction is often sufficient to eliminate obstruction (Johnston 1969) but, with the exception of some cases of persistent fetal folds, the angulations reform post-operatively so that some form of pyeloplasty is nearly always needed. In the great majority of cases of hydronephrosis in children dismembered pyeloureterostomy of the Anderson-Hynes (1963) type is applicable (Fig. 8.3). For obstruction associated with an aberrant renal artery, the anastomosis is performed anterior to the vessel. Because of the small size of the ureter in young children and infants it is the author's practice to splint the anastomosis and perform nephrostomy routinely. There has been no significant resulting infection and the small risk of its occurrence seems preferable to disruption of the suture line due to obstructive post-operative oedema and the possible consequences of healing by second intention, peri-pelvic fibrosis and subsequent secondary obstruction.

Pelviureteric obstruction in a malrotated kidney such as a horseshoe or an ectopic pelvic kidney is usually associated with a high ureteric insertion on a high-sited pelvis. In such cases the standard dismembered operation may not allow the construction of a funnel-shaped pelvis coning straight into the ureter. Correction of the malrotation, which with a horseshoe kidney necessitates division of the renal bridge, may improve the anatomical arrangement but often it is prevented by an anomalous renal blood supply. A simpler, and equally effective technique is the pelvic flap pyeloplasty of Culp and Deweerd (1951), which allows the formation of a dependent pelviureteric junction without the need to alter the position of the kidney.

Results

Pyeloureteroplasty for hydronephrosis in children produces excellent clinical results in that morbidity is minimal, complications are very uncommon and symptoms are generally entirely relieved. However, the pyelographic appearance after surgery is often disappointing in that the calyceal outlines rarely return to normal except in early or intermittently obstructed cases. Johnston et al. (1977) evaluated 140 kidneys by pyelography before and after pyeloureteroplasty and noted at follow up that calyceal dilatation had lessened in 82, was unchanged in 53 and in 5 had increased. Isotope methods give a more favourable impression of the results of surgery. Johnston and Kathel (1972) compared pre- and post-operative isotope renograms assessed by analogue computer simulation from 32 hydronephrotic kidneys in children. Even when the pyelograms before and after surgery were similar, 23 kidneys were found to have improved tubular function and 29 had increased emptying rates following pyeloureteroplasty (see Chap. 4).

References

Anderson JC (1963) Hydronephrosis. Heinemann, London

Bratt CG, Aurell M, Nilsson S (1977) Renal function in patients with hydronephrosis. Br J Urol 49: 249–252

Cohen B, Geldman SM, Kopilnick M, Khwana AV, Salik JO (1978) Ureteropelvic junction ωstruction: Its occurrence in three members of a single family. J Urol 120: 361–363

Culp OS, Deweerd JH (1951) A pelvic flap operation for certain types of ureteropelvic obstruction. Mayo Clin Proc 26: 483–485

Foote JW, Blennerhasset JB, Wiglesworth FW, Mackinson KJ (1970) Observation on the ureteropelvic junction. J Urol 104: 252–255

Johnston JH (1969) The pathogenesis of hydronephrosis in childhood. Br J Urol 41: 724–728

Johnston JH, Kathel BL (1972) The results of surgery for hydronephrosis as determined by renography with analogue computer simulation. Br J Urol 44: 320–325

Johnston JH, Evans JP, Glassberg KI, Shapiro SR (1977) Pelvic hydronephrosis in children. A review of 219 personal cases. J Urol 117: 97–102

Matz LR, Craven JD, Hodson CJ (1969) Experimental obstructive nephropathy in the pig. II. Pathology. Br J Urol 41 [Suppl]

Mirandi D, De Assis AS (1975) Transitional cell papilloma of ureter in young boy. Urology 5: 559

Murnaghan GF (1958) The dynamics of the renal pelvis and ureter with reference to congenital hydronephrosis. Br J Urol 30: 321–325

Notley RG (1968) Electron microscopy of the upper ureter and the pelviureteric junction. Br J Urol 40: 37–40

Robson WJ, Rudy SM, Johnston JH (1976) Pelviureteric obstruction in infancy. J Pediatr Surg 11: 57–60

Vaughan ED, Buhler FR, Laragh JH (1974) Normal renin secretion in hypertensive patients with primarily unilateral chronic hydronephrosis. J Urol 112: 153–155

Whitaker RH (1975) Some observations and theories on the wide ureter and hydronephrosis. Br J Urol 47: 377–381

Williams DI, Karlaftis CM (1966) Hydronephrosis due to pelviureteric obstruction in the newborn. Br J Urol 38: 138–141

Winterburn MH, France NE (1972) Arterial changes associated with hydronephrosis in infants and children. Br J Urol 44: 96–100

9.   The Role of Percutaneous Nephrostomy

R.C. Pfister

This chapter deals with nephrostomy and other percutaneous procedures (drainage of perirenal fluid collections, dilatation of stenosis, stone dissolution, calculus extraction) which are applicable in the therapeutic and diagnostic management of obstruction at the pelviureteric junction.

Temporary percutaneous nephrostomy (PCN) is an important addition to the urologic armamentarium. Initially described as a diagnostic test of residual function in unilateral chronic renal obstruction (Goodwin et al. 1955), the procedure has evolved as the method of choice for emergency drainage of the obstructed upper urinary tract in those medical centres where the technique is available (Stables et al. 1978). In many institutions, it has replaced conventional surgical pyelostomy and retrograde catheterisation for establishing drainage of an obstructed kidney.

Pelviureteric junction (PUJ) malfunction constitutes an important cause of obstructive nephropathy. While there has been considerable controversy regarding the mechanism of the pathogenesis of this type of hydronephrosis, the aetiologic puzzle is beginning to be solved as attested by the discussions elsewhere in this book.

At the Massachusetts General Hospital 314 percutaneous nephrostomies on 287 adult and pediatric kidneys have been performed. They were employed 27 times in 26 patients (20 adults and six children) with PUJ problems. The obstruction was congenital (idiopathic) in 20 kidneys and acquired in six (Table 9.1).

Table 9.1. Percutaneous procedures in pelviureteric junction obstruction

	No. of patients
Renal Drainage (Nephrostomy)	
Sepsis (pyonephrosis 9)	11
Anuria	3
Pain	3
Split function	4
Fallout of surgical nephrostomy tube	2
Leak postoperative	3
	26
Other Techniques	
Retroperitoneal drainage (perirenal abscess 2, urinoma 1)	3
Stone dissolution (struvite)	1
Stone extraction (oxalate)	1
Dilatation of operative stenosis	2
	7

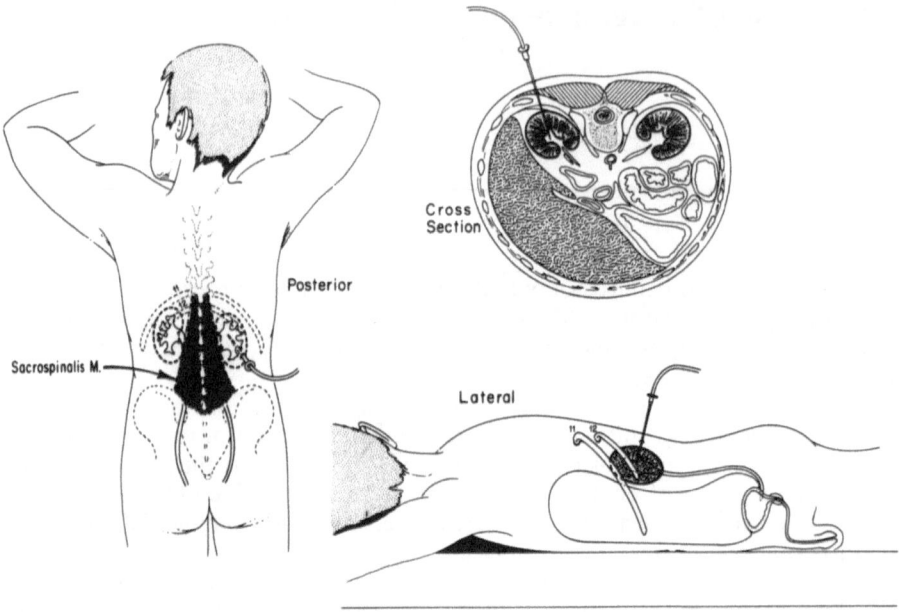

Fig. 9.1. Schema for percutaneous pyelography with 22g needle. Note needle passage below the 12th rib to avoid causing pneumothorax. From: Radiol Clin North Am 1979, 17: 341.

Technique

The initial procedure performed is percutaneous antegrade pyelography (Fig. 9.1). Here, the term is restricted to its use in (a) determining opening/resting pressure, (b) obtaining renal pelvic urine for analysis or (c) injecting contrast media to evaluate anatomy or demonstrate pathology (Pfister and Newhouse 1979a,b; Pfister et al. 1978). The aspirated urine may be subjected to (1) biochemical analysis, (2) cytologic evaluation or (3) smears and cultures to identify bacteria, fungi or acid-fast organisms. Cloudy urine suggests pyonephrosis and immediate antibiotic therapy with percutaneous drainage is indicated to obviate septicemic shock.

In infants and younger children, sedation[1] is helpful in relieving anxiety and the sensation of local pressure during the placement of large catheters in the kidney or perirenal space during local anaesthesia. Neither heavy sedation nor general anaesthesia is needed or desirable.

Fluoroscopic guidance is required for proper positioning of the catheter and standard radiography for documentation of the upper urinary tract and its surrounding tissue. Neither ultrasound (Pedersen et al. 1976) nor computerised tomography (Haaga et al. 1977) offer enough help to outweigh their disadvantages (Stables et al. 1978).

Two basic techniques (angiographic and trocar) have been developed for percutaneous catheterisation of the kidney and/or perirenal area.

[1]Mixture of merperidine 25 mg, promethazine 5 mg and chlorpromazine 8 mg. (Dose of 1 ml/25 lb should not exceed 2 ml.)

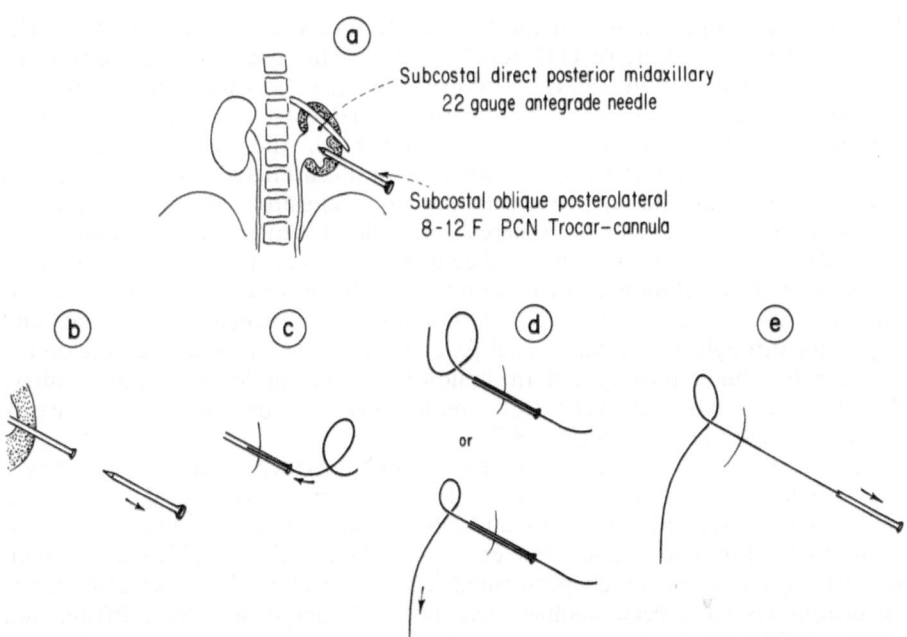

Fig. 9.2. Schema for trocar percutaneous nephrostomy following antegrade pyelography. A more lateral position of the drainage catheter provides greater patient comfort when lying supine. From: Radiol Clin North Am 1979, 17: 351.

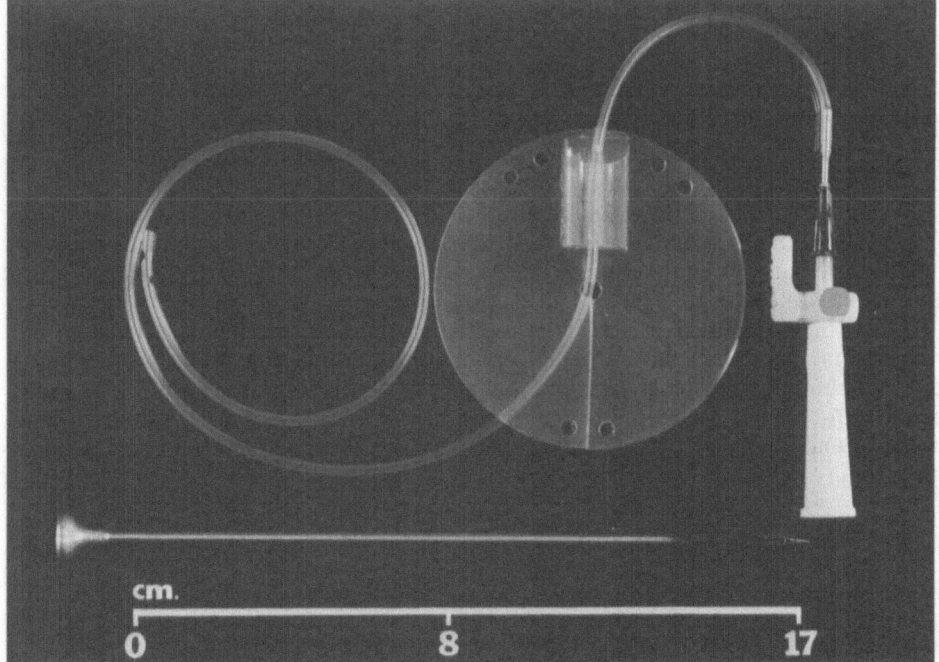

Fig. 9.3. Percutaneous nephrostomy equipment. Prototype trocar-cannula unit is long enough to reach those kidneys at maximum depth. Soft silicone catheter is anchored to plastic holder on the skin; blunt-ended needle, 3-way stopcock, and flange are taped to a padded tongue blade for fixation.

The modified angiographic method of PCN involves the passage of a stiff guidewire through a needle or catheter-sheathed needle, dilatation of the tract by successive vascular teflon dilators before the final introduction of a firm angiographic-type catheter or a balloon catheter (Burnett et al. 1976). J-shaped guidewires and pigtailed catheters are desirable for the Seldinger technique. However, except in the infant, the kidney is several centimeters from the skin and the renal parenchyma has a propensity for rapid closure. The guidewire has a tendency to tear or fragment the tapered and coiled tip of the angiographic PCN catheter. Many workers find the method cumbersome and extensively manipulative.

As an alternative technique, trocar-cannula units have been utilised for PCN. The trocar has a smooth pencil-point tip without cutting edges which promotes safe and easy passage through the vascular renal parenchyma. The recessed side hole on the trocar permits a fluid return through the hollow bore which indicates successful entry. Following trocar removal, very soft non-kinking silicone catheters are easily advanced through the cannula (Fig. 9.2).

Such prototype PCN units have facilitated rapid placement of drainage catheters (5 Fr—infant, 8 Fr—children, 12 Fr—adult) into the pelvicalyceal system and retroperitoneal space (Fig. 9.3). In addition, other procedures such as ureteral stenting, ureteral dilatation and stone extraction via a 10 Fr steerable catheter with stone basket can be immediately performed. The technical details of performance of these procedures have been detailed elsewhere (Dretler et al. 1979; Pfister and Newhouse 1979 a, b).

Materials

In 26 patients there were 27 PCNs performed with one kidney undergoing catheter placement on separate occasions two years apart (pre- and post-pyeloplasty). Three patients had another catheter placed percutaneously in the retroperitoneal space to drain a simultaneous fluid collection (perirenal abscess, urinoma).

In addition to PCN, three kidneys underwent four additional procedures. Dilatation of the PUJ area was performed in two urinary tracts which had previous renal pelvic surgery with resulting stricture. One of these systems also had stone extraction while another kidney had dissolution of a stone.

Pain in the flank, back or abdomen was the commonest complaint in twelve of the patients; nine had high intrapelvicalyceal pressures and three of these were anuric, one had abdominal distension from a large tense perirenal urinoma following renal pelvic surgery and anastomotic leak; one had pyonephrosis with unmeasurable pressure and another patient had a recurrent non-obstructing stone and urinary infection.

Renal Drainage

Sepsis with high fever (sometimes with hypotension and bacteraemia) was the presenting symptom in 11 patients, and frank pus (pyonephrosis) was present in nine kidneys at the time of PCN. Two of the pyonephroses were a result of fungal

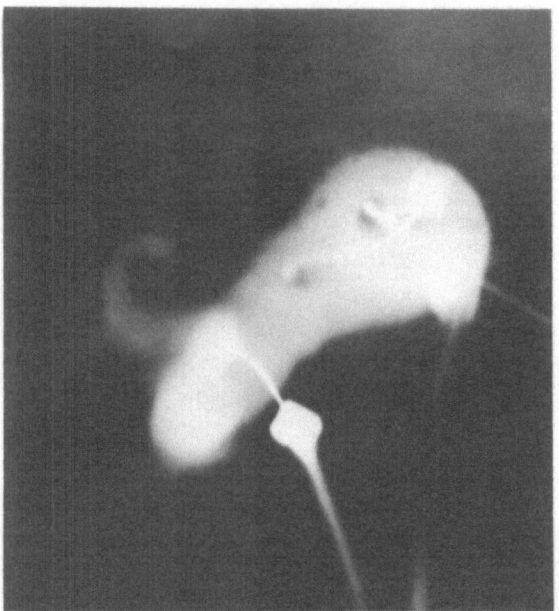

Fig. 9.4. Percutaneous pyelography and nephrostomy in 82-year-old female diabetic patient with sepsis and fungal pyonephrosis (Candidiasis) in PUJ obstruction. From: Am J Roentgenol 1977, 129: 415.

infection (candidiasis, torulopsis) with bacteria-free urine and no previous antibiotic treatment. Both patients were diabetics and one died within a week from cardiac consequences of the infection (Fig. 9.4), (Dembner and Pfister 1977). The other patients survived, with PCN having played a crucial role in their initial management by allowing time for treatment of sepsis and shock. The subsequent pyeloplasty or nephrectomy was then performed on a sterile kidney.

Severe azotaemia was present in three patients and was associated with anuria and a solitary kidney in each case. One patient had recurrent moderate deterioration of renal function two years following apparent successful pyeloplasty. Two percutaneous ureteral perfusion studies were normal (differential pressure below 12 cmH$_2$O) during this interval and a second period of PCN drainage for three weeks did not alter renal function; the catheter was then removed (Fig. 9.5).

Four kidneys had split renal function studies following PCN. In two cases they were the primary reason for PCN and in the others they were done subsequent to decompression for pain or pyonephrosis. Determination of individual renal function remains a valid reason for PCN since radionuclide studies may not accurately predict recoverability of renal function in the obstructed kidney.

In two cases, replacement of surgical nephrostomy tubes (inserted during pyeloplasty) were unsuccessful. Attempts to re-enter the kidney under flouroscopic control also failed since some hours had passed and the original nephrostomy tract in the renal parenchyma had closed. Both kidneys required PCN through the original cutaneous site but with a new renal puncture location.

In two pediatric kidneys 5 Fr polyethylene catheters (flexible naso-gastric tubes) were used; in the other children and all adults 8–12 Fr soft silicone catheters were used for PCN drainage. In one instance a modified angiographic PCN technique was used; in all others trocar PCN was employed.

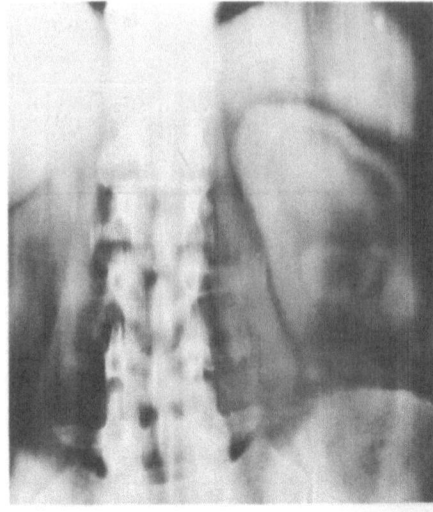

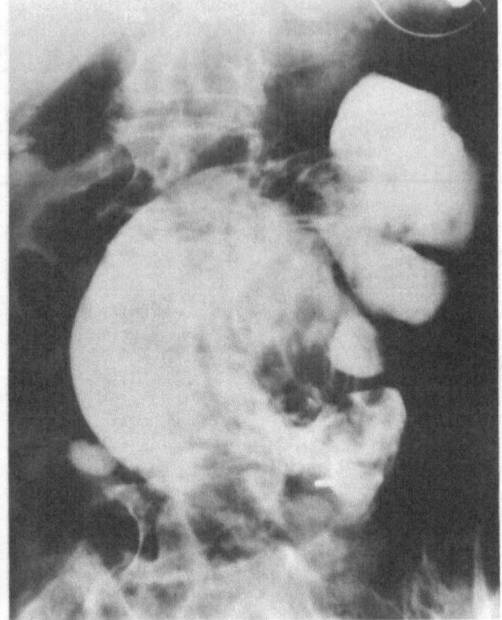

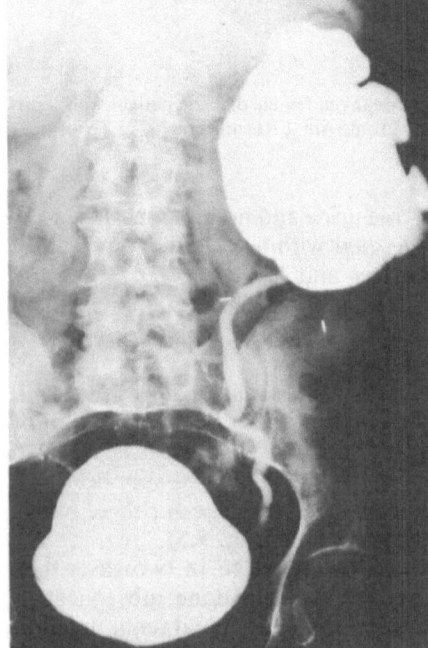

Fig. 9.5. A 68-year-old female patient presented with flank pain and anuria. **a** Nephrotomography reveals solitary hypertrophied kidney (22 cm long) with caliectasis. **b** High-grade congenital PUJ obstruction; numerous blood clots from 3 unit bleed within the pyelocalyceal system following percutaneous nephrostomy. **c** Two years after pyeloplasty mild azotemia developed; normal needle perfusion studies were verified by lack of improvement in renal function with drainage from a second percutaneous nephrostomy (uneventful).

Retroperitoneal Drainage

Urinary leaks occurred in three cases within the first week, in two following renal pelvic lithotomy and in the third after lithotomy with pyeloplasty. In two cases, PUJ obstruction developed— in one of these a large perirenal urinoma appeared to be responsible. Since elevated intrapelvic pressure stresses the anastomosis and increases urine extravasation, painful abdominal distension and fever results. Percutaneous catheter placement into the perirenal urinoma controls the pain.

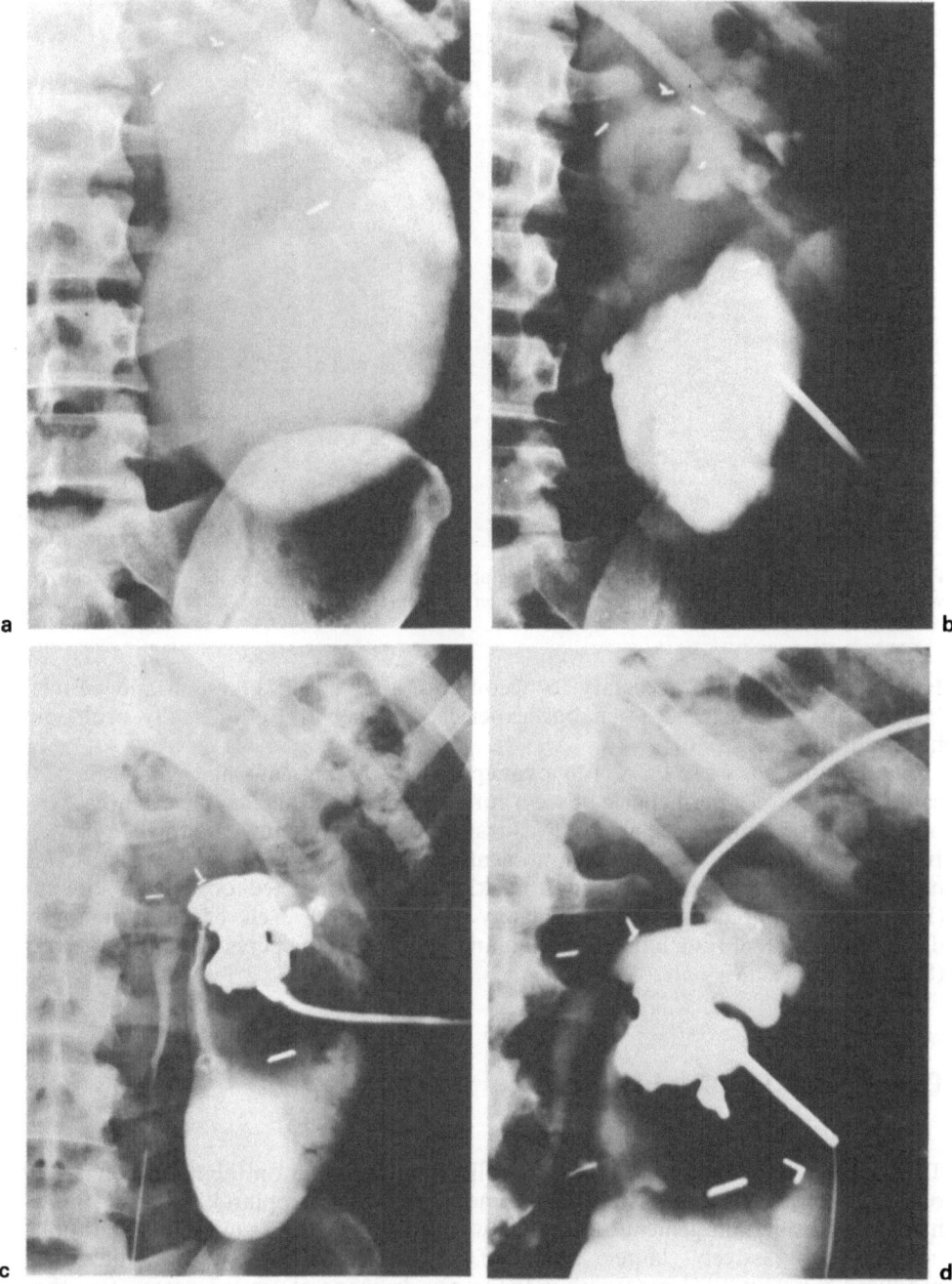

Fig. 9.6. Fever, pain, and abdominal distension developed in a 27-year-old man following pyelolithotomy and an apparent acquired PUJ obstruction. **a** Urography showing dense accumulation of contrast media in kidney and perirenal space. **b** Percutaneous catheterisation of the urinoma; opening pressure of 28 cmH$_2$O and cloudy urine. The retroperitoneal catheter drained 1500 ml of urine per 24 hours for 5 days; but **c** the leak from the renal pelvis persisted and **d** concomitant percutaneous nephrostomy was performed to manage this problem.

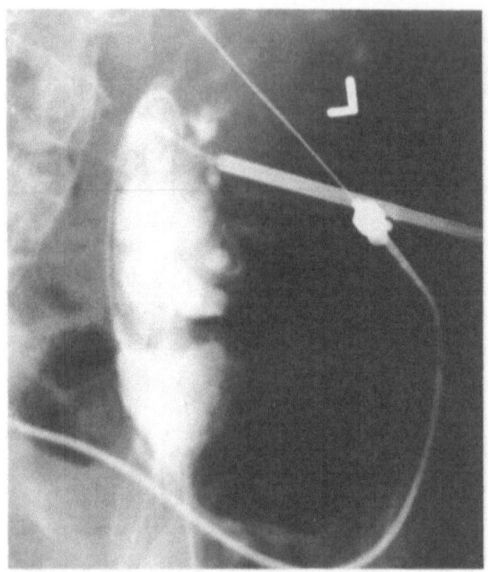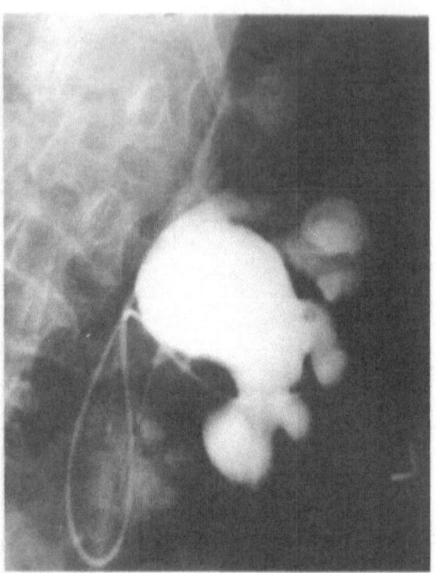

a   b

Fig. 9.7. Simultaneous drainage of a perinephric abscess (**a**) and pyonephrosis (**b**) rescued an elderly woman with bacteraemia and hypotension from her congenital PUJ obstruction. From: Radiol Clin North Am 1979, 17: 351.

However, PCN is also necessary to decompress the collecting system and permit healing of the anastomosis; in our experience, delay in PCN usually prolongs hospitalisation (Fig. 9.6).

In conjunction with PCN for pyonephrosis two patients had percutaneous catheterisation of a perinephric abscess for concomitant drainage of both areas. In one, a renal transplant, the abscess was transrenal and communicated with a calyx. In the other patient no calyceal communication was shown and the perirenal abscess may have resulted from pyelosinus backflow in the infected obstructed kidney (Fig. 9.7). Nephrectomy was ultimately performed in each because of total diminution of renal function rather than any inability of the percutaneous catheters (8–12 Fr) to drain.

Dilatation of Operative PUJ Strictures

Two kidneys developed PUJ strictures following operation on the renal pelvis. In one case obstruction persisted for 3 months after pyeloplasty for congenital hydronephrosis. Enlargement of the PUJ was accomplished as a one-time dilatation utilising progressively larger semi-stiff catheters. The resulting dilatation produced a patent PUJ area with satisfactory drainage at least 2 years after the procedure.

In the other patient a long segment of narrowing in the upper ureter developed after a pyelolithotomy leak. Weeks later, after stone extraction, a series of dilating external stent catheter exchanges were made over several weeks (Fig. 9.8) (Pingoud et al. 1980). After catheter removal, subsequent urography showed further

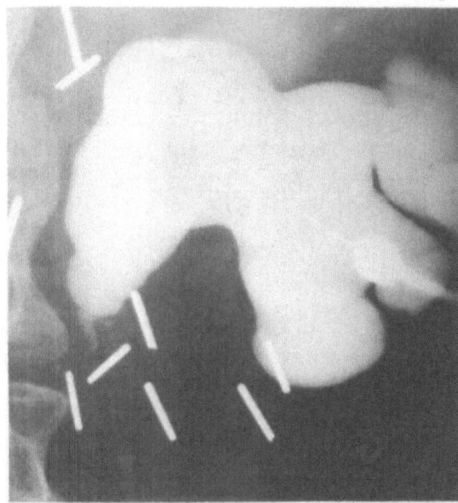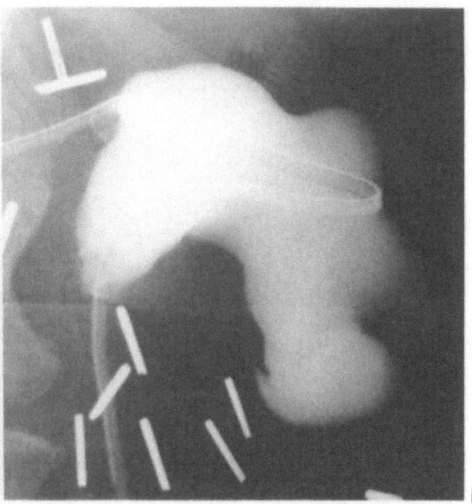

a

b

Fig. 9.8. **a** Percutaneous ureteral perfusion some weeks following pyelolithotomy and leak; acquired PUJ obstruction, upper ureteral stenosis and high differential pressures (25 cmH$_2$O). **b** Percutaneous dilatation with series of external stent catheters; the final 10 Fr tube was not advanced far enough down the ureter and healing incorporated the side holes in the catheter tip, which avulsed during subsequent removal.

hydronephrosis. At exploration, the tip of the final dilating catheter was found embedded in the urothelium; unrecognised avulsion or separation of the catheter in the upper ureter had occurred during removal.

Stone Dissolution

Complete dissolution of a struvite pyelocalyceal stone was accomplished in one case following irrigation of an acidic solvent (Renacidin) through a PCN catheter (Dretler et al. 1979). This kidney had a previous pyeloplasty and pyelolithotomy for triple phosphate calculus. A percutaneous ureteral perfusion study was initially performed which indicated there was no obstruction in the upper urinary tract. A single PCN catheter was then placed for irrigation at low pressures after antibiotics had rendered the urine sterile (Fig. 9.9). Further details on non-operative management of urinary calculi have been described elsewhere (Smith et al. 1978; Spataro et al. 1978) (Fig. 9.10).

Stone Extraction

Percutaneous extraction of retained stones was performed on one kidney following pyelolithotomy for innumerable calculi. A steerable catheter with stone basket was utilised for the removal of the remaining two stones through a nephrostomy tract

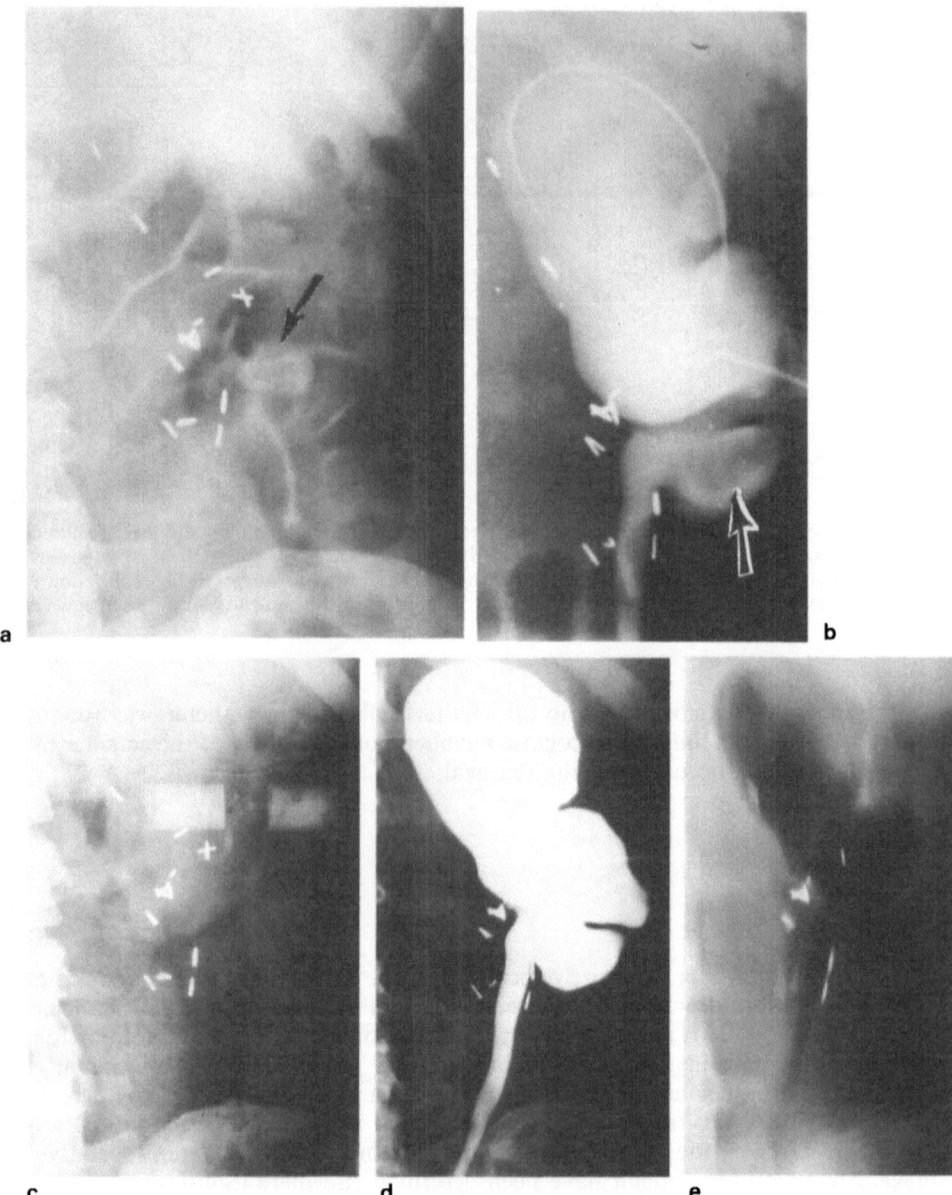

Fig. 9.9. Twenty-four-year-old woman with urinary tract infection and recurrent lower calyceal stone; previous pyelolithotomy and pyeloplasty. **a** Plain film and **b** percutaneous nephrostomy (note stone; *arrows*). Following irrigation for a struvite-calculus the plain film (**c**) positive-contrast (**d**) and negative-contrast (air) (**e**) pyelograms indicate complete stone dissolution.

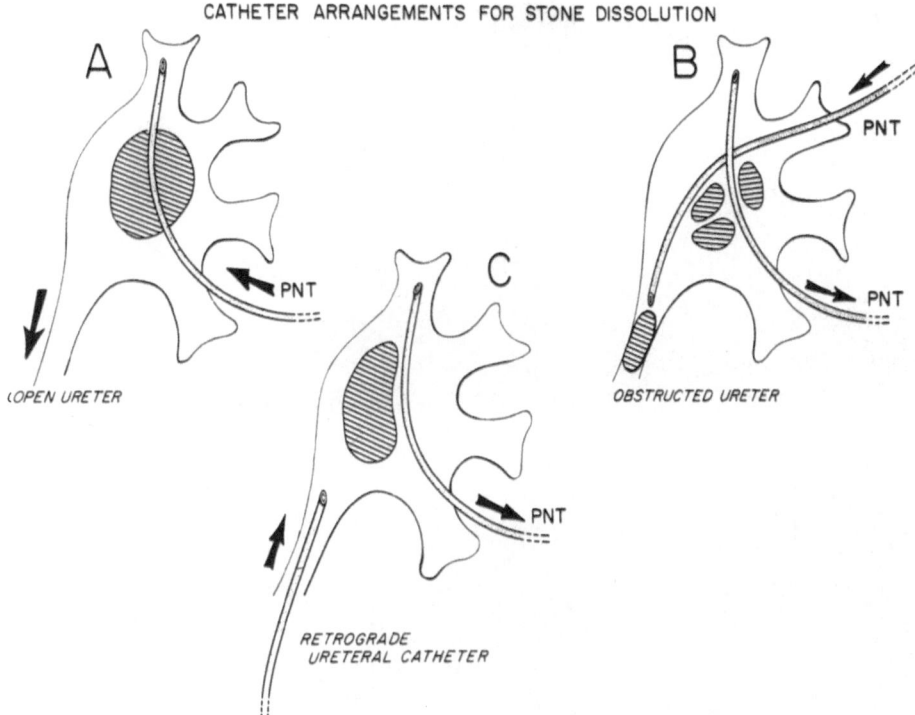

Fig. 9.10. Schema of potential catheter arrangements for low-pressure solvent irrigation during dissolution of a calculus. From: New Engl J Med 1979, 300: 341.

under fluoroscopic control (Fig. 9.11). The procedure and equipment (Fig. 9.12) is similar to that used for biliary stone removal and is preferred to stone grasping forceps (Fernstrom and Johansson 1976; Palestrant et al. 1980).

Complications

Complications resulting from interventional percutaneous procedures occurred in three patients; some are correctable. A PCN tube (5 Fr) placed in a young child did not drain properly due to inadequate size of the side holes placed in the tube. In another case a retained catheter fragment remained within the ureteral segment undergoing dilatation. The distal side holes of the dilating stent catheter had not been advanced far enough beyond the injured portion of ureter and they became firmly incorporated within the regenerated urothelial lining. In the third complication, haemorrhage occurred within the pyelocalyceal system which required transfusion of three units of blood; at surgery the extrarenal space was free of haematoma.

No percutaneously placed catheter fell out in this series of patients and a sutured anchoring plastic disc holding the PCN tube has been advantageous in this regard.

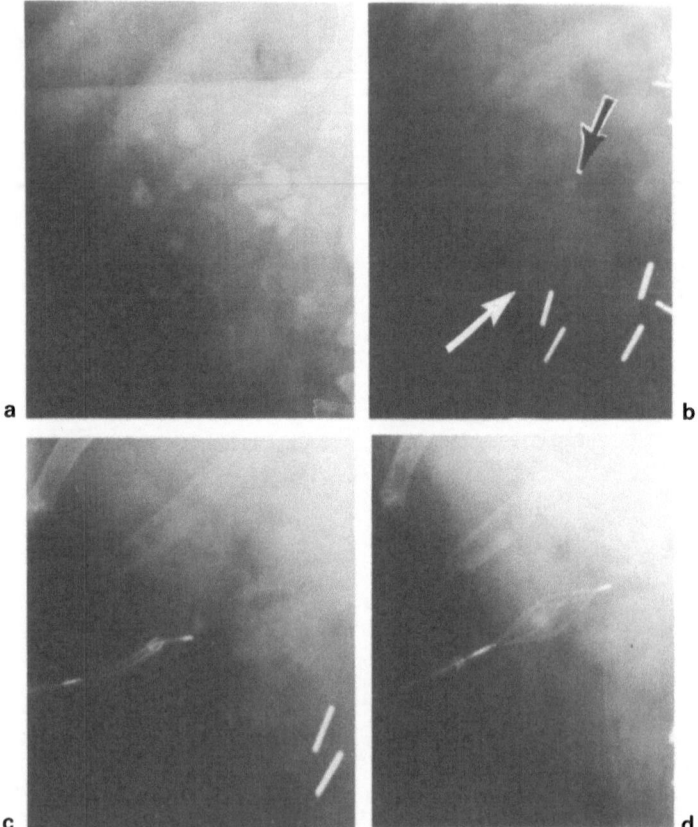

Fig. 9.11. Plain radiographs demonstrating **a** over 20 stones in the kidney and **b** two retained calculi (*arrows*) following nephrolithotomy. **c** Guided catheter with Dormia basket positioned near one stone. **d** The engaged stone was extraced via a nephrostomy tract.

Summary

In this series, 33% of patients with PUJ obstruction had pyonephrosis. In many of the others anuria, postoperative urine leak, accidental loss of surgical nephrostomy tube and postoperative pain posed significant problems. In such cases, urgent percutaneous drainage may save the kidney and even the patient's life.

Following nephrostomy, other procedures can be undertaken which are both deliberate and planned. Thus, split renal function determination, dilatation of operative strictures and stone extraction or dissolution are also possible using this technique.

Acknowledgements. The author wishes to acknowledge the help and cooperation he has received during this study from the following colleagues: Dr W. Hardy Hendren, Dr Jefferey H. Newhouse, Dr George R. Prout Jr, Dr Isobel Yoder and Dr Niall M. Heney.

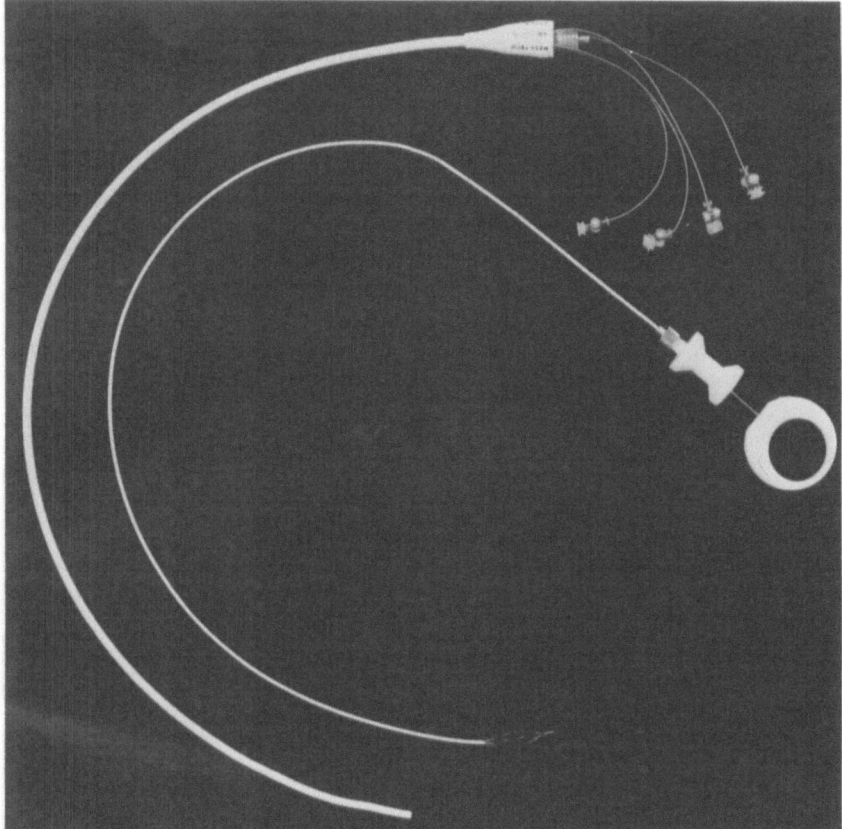

Fig. 9.12. Equipment for percutaneous pyeloureteral stone removal. *Above,* 10 Fr Steerable catheter (handle not shown); *below,* stone basket.

References

Burnett LL, Correa RJ Jr, Bush WH Jr (1976) A new method for percutaneous nephrostomy. Radiology 120: 557–561

Dembner AG, Pfister RC (1977) Fungal infection of the urinary tract: Demonstration by antegrade pyelography and drainage by percutaneous nephrostomy. Am J Roentgenol 129: 415–418

Dretler SP, Pfister RC, Newhouse JH (1979) Renal stone dissolution via percutaneous nephrostomy. N Engl J Med 300: 341–343

Fernstrom I, Johansson B (1976) Percutaneous pyelolithotomy: A new extraction technique. Scand J Urol Nephrol 10: 257–259

Goodwin WE, Casey WC, Wolf W (1955) Percutaneous trocar (needle) nephrostomy in hydronephrosis. JAMA 157: 891–899

Haaga JR, Zelch MG, Alfidi RJ, Stewart BH, Daugherty JD (1977) CT-guided antegrade pyelography and percutaneous nephrostomy. Am J Roentgenol 128: 621–624

Palestrant AM, Rad FF, Sacks BA, Klein LA (1980) Postoperative percutaneous kidney stone extraction. Radiology 134: 778–779

Pedersen JF, Cowan DF, Kristensen JK, Holm HH, Hancke S, Jensen F (1976) Ultrasonically-guided percutaneous nephrostomy. Radiology 119: 429–431

Pfister RC, Newhouse JH (1979a) Interventional percutaneous pyeloureteral techniques. I. Antegrade pyelography and ureteral perfusion. Radiol Clin North Am 17: 341–350

Pfister RC, Newhouse JH (1979b) Percutaneous nephrostomy and other procedures. Radiol Clin North Am 17: 351-363

Pfister RC, Newhouse JH, Yoder IC (1978) Applications of a renal trocarcannula unit. Am J Roentgenol 130: 584

Pingoud EG, Bagley DH, Deman RK, Glancy KE, Pais OS (1980) Percutaneous antegrade bilateral ureteral dilatation and stent placement for internal drainage. Radiology 134: 780

Smith AD, Lange PH, Miller RP, Reinke DB (1979) Dissolution of cystine calculi by irrigation with acetylcysteine through percutaneous nephrostomy. Urology 13: 422-423

Spataro RF, Linke CA, Barbaric ZL (1978) The use of percutaneous nephrostomy and urinary alkalinization in the dissolution of obstructing uric acid stones. Radiology 129: 629-632

Stables DB, Ginsberg NJ, Johnson ML (1978) Percutaneous nephrostomy: A series and review of the literature. Am J Roentgenol 130: 75-82

10. Clinical Management

S.A. Koff

Idiopathic hydronephrosis is primarily a radiographic diagnosis made by recognition on the intravenous urogram (IVU) of an enlarged pelvicalyceal system. Successful management depends not only on diagnosis, but also on determining the aetiology and significance of the dilatation and then instituting appropriate therapy. Until recently, the demonstration of hydronephrosis was usually considered presumptive evidence for pelviureteric junction obstruction and diagnosis was followed by corrective surgery. This approach was predicated on the assumption that hydronephrosis was due to obstruction and was invariably progressive throughout life (Roberts and Slade 1964). Such a supposition, however, has never been proven and recent evidence suggests that it may not be true for a significant number of patients. Firstly, it is now well appreciated that hydronephrosis does not necessarily equate with obstruction because a variety of congenital, acquired and postoperative conditions have been observed to produce pelvicalyceal dilatation and to simulate obstruction in its absence (Whitaker 1978). Further, the changes of hydronephrosis on the IVP are merely a chronicle of prior morphologic alterations which have affected the kidney but do not define obstruction or indicate the likelihood for progressive renal deterioration (Djurhuus et al. 1976; Wax and McDonald 1966). Secondly, as assessed by renography, clearance techniques and urinary concentrating ability, many patients with genuine hydronephrosis have no measurable reduction in renal parenchymal function (Bratt et al. 1977; Nilsson et al. 1979). Thirdly, conservative (non-operative) management of selected patients with hydronephrosis has resulted neither in diminution of renal function nor in progressive urinary tract dilatation (Bratt et al. 1977). Finally, the reported results of corrective pelviureteric surgery with respect to IVP appearances and renal function, although varying considerably from series to series, have been often less than ideal with up to 40% of patients showing no measurable postoperative improvement (Drake et al. 1978; Johnston et al. 1977; Hendren et al. 1980; Williams and Kenaw 1976).

These findings suggest that certain patients with hydronephrosis either have no demonstrable obstruction or have a mild degree of obstruction which has reached a state of equilibrium such that progression of disease may not occur (Hoyt 1954). This situation has important therapeutic implications because surgical intervention in these instances would not be needed or beneficial. As a consequence, the diagnosis of hydronephrosis cannot be considered complete nor can rational therapeutic decisions be made until the functional significance of the suspected obstruction is assessed fully (Whitaker 1977; Kreuger et al. 1980).

The major impediment to the complete evaluation of hydronephrosis has been a frustrating inability to precisely define obstruction in the partially obstructed urinary tract. This is because in partial urinary tract obstruction the usual physiological parameters for characterising obstruction (such as elevated pressure and reduced flow rate) are not usually, if at all, abnormal. Likewise, the conventional methods for investigating hydronephrosis (such as the IVU, standard renography and ultrasound) neither determine whether or not obstruction exists nor predict which dilated system will improve after surgery. The experimental canine studies described in Chap. 7 suggested that partial obstruction may be defined on the basis of intrarenal pelvic pressure-volume changes which occur during volume expansion; however, that methodology is currently not applicable for routine clinical use.

Although considerable experience has been accumulated using the newer diagnostic methods of assessing obstruction, their application to the overall management of patients with idiopathic hydronephrosis has not yet been completely explored, at least prospectively. Because most patients who are identified as having truly significant obstruction usually undergo surgery, clinical studies comparable to the preceding canine investigations may not be feasible. It would be extremely informative, however, to examine prospectively the fate of patients with genuine hydronephrosis who are identified as having no significant obstruction and who, consequently, do not have corrective surgery.

The following study was undertaken during the past few years. Perfusion pressure flow measurements and diuresis renography were used to assess the significance of suspected pelviureteric junction obstructions. The study examines the impact of these diagnostic tools on the overall management of patients with hydronephrosis and presents prospective data on the fate of patients assessed as having no obstruction and who did not undergo surgical treatment.

Clinical Material

From 1976 to 1980, 82 patients (36 adults and 46 children) were evaluated at the University of Michigan Medical Center for idiopathic hydronephrosis and suspected pelviureteric junction obstruction. The age and sex incidence and the side of the

Table 10.1. Sex and age indicence and side affected

	No. of patients
Sex	
Male	49
Female	33
Age	
0–5	22
6–18	24
19–40	17
40–60	12
> 60	7
Laterality	
Right	36
Left	40
Bilateral	6

Table 10.2. Presenting clinical features

	No. of patients
Pain	45
Increasing with fluid, 3	
Haematuria	14
Following mild trauma, 4	
Urinary tract infection	14
Abdominal mass	17
Uraemia	2
Hypertension	2
Asymptomatic	14

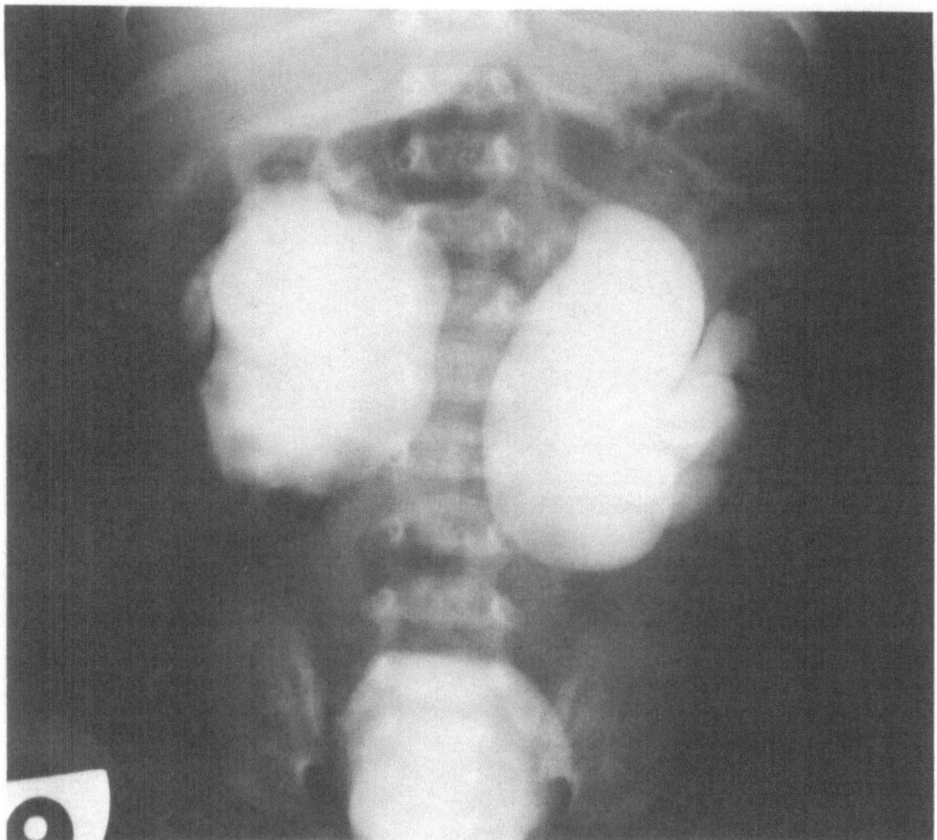

Fig. 10.1.   Bilateral ureteropelvic junction obstruction presenting in infancy.

hydronephrosis are shown in Table 10.1. The presenting signs and symptoms are listed in Table 10.2. Pain, haematuria and urinary infection were more common in older children and adults while infants usually presented with an abdominal mass. Fourteen patients were totally asymptomatic; 13 were adults (mean age = 61 years) and hydronephrosis was discovered during investigations for unrelated conditions.

Intravenous urography (IVU) demonstrated typical findings of pelviureteric junction obstruction— pelvicalyceal dilatation with parenchymal thinning— in 69 kidneys (Fig. 10.1). In 12 cases massive dilatation and/or non-visualisation occurred while in five, large extrarenal pelves with minimal calyceal changes were noted. Calculi within the calyces or parenchymal calcifications were observed in 12 patients all of whom had no detectable metabolic abnormalities. Calculi composition was calcium oxalate or phosphate and no patient had a staghorn calculus or a stone in the renal pelvis which might cause obstruction. Associated congenital genitourinary tract anomalies occurred in 18% of patients and are recorded in Table 10.3. Three children with hydronephrosis and ipsilateral grade 3-4 reflux are included because each presented with an abdominal mass, two had solitary kidneys and one was anuric and uraemic.

Voiding cystography was used to exclude reflux in 19 children. Ultrasound identified hydronephrosis in seven instances and antegrade pyelography established

Table 10.3. Associated genitourinary tract
anomalies

	No. of patients
Contralateral lesion	9
Multicystic kidney, 2	
Renal agenesis, 4	
Obstructed megaureter, 1	
Vesicoureteral reflux, 2	
Horseshoe kidney	1
Pelvic kidney	2
Bladder diverticula	1
Ipsilateral vesicoureteral reflux	3

Table 10.4. Diagnostic methods for assessing hydronephrosis

	No. of patients	
Perfusion pressure flow		
Pre-operative		13
$p > 23\,cmH_2O$	11	
$p < 20\,cmH_2O$	2	
Post-operative		5
$p < 18\,cmH_2O$	4	
$p = 22\,cmH_2O$	1	
Diuresis renography		
Initial		33
Obstruction	20	
No obstruction	10	
Poor function	3	
Early post-operative (< 2 weeks)		15
No obstruction	13	
Poor function	2	
Late post-operative		25
No obstruction	22	
Obstruction	2	
False obstruction	1	

the diagnosis in two patients with non-visualised kidneys on IVP. In 37 patients, retrograde ureterograms were performed to prove that the ureter was of normal calibre.

Perfusion pessure flow studies were used in 13 patients; 12 were intra-operative studies and one was as an outpatient. Pressures were greater than $23\,cmH_2O$ in 11 patients and less than $20\,cmH_2O$ in two patients who showed clinical improvement after pyeloplasty. Postoperative perfusion examination in five patients revealed pressures less than $10\,cmH_2O$ in four and a value of $22\,cmH_2O$ in one (Table 10.4).

Diuresis renography was performed pre-operatively in 25 patients. Obstruction was identified in 20, all of whom showed radiographic improvement after

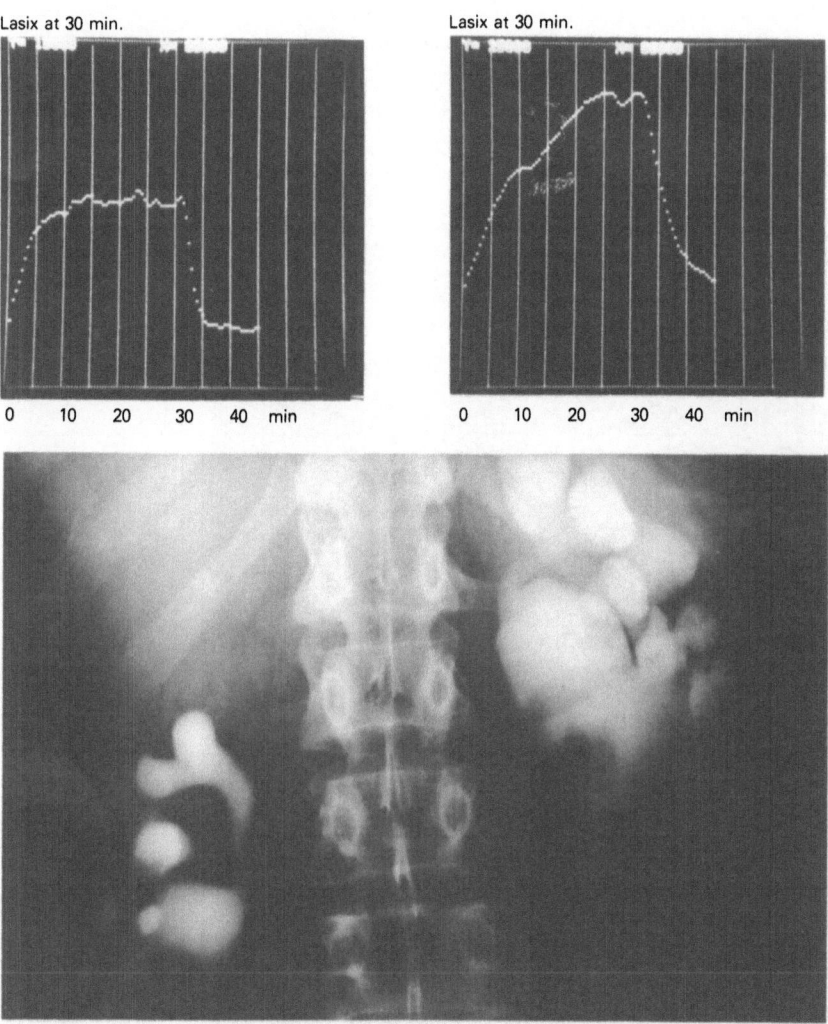

Fig. 10.2. Diuresis renography evaluation for idiopathic hydronephrosis with suspected left ureteropelvic junction obstruction demonstrates the dilated but non-obstructed pattern in both kidneys.

pyeloplasty. In two cases with intermittent flank pain, the studies were performed in the absence of pain and obstruction was not noted. The remaining three cases had such poor renal function that no assessment of obstruction was possible (Table 10.4).

Eight other patients studied by diuresis renography showed no evidence of obstruction (Fig. 10.2). No operation was performed on these patients and none has since required corrective surgery. Six of these patients were asymptomatic and two had intermittent flank pain.

Diuresis renography was used to assess the results of surgery in 40 patients (Fig. 10.3). In 15 cases the examination was performed in the early postoperative period (within 14 days of pyeloplasty); 13 patients displayed a non-obstructed pattern which was corroborated by follow-up IVP, while in two cases severe functional impairment prevented evaluation. Late follow-up examinations (6 months to 4

Lasix at 15 min.

Lasix at 15 min.

0   5   10   15   20   25   30

0   5   10   15   20   25   30

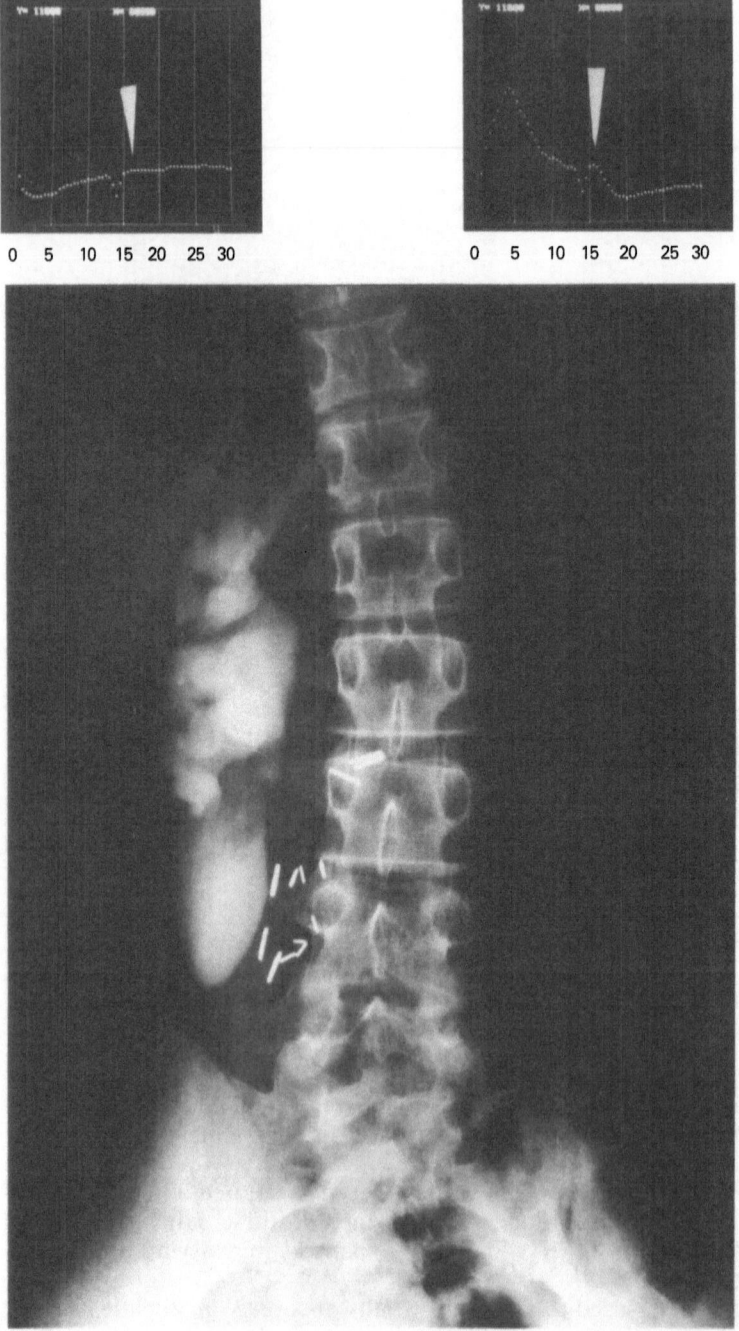

a

Fig. 10.3. Early postoperative assessment of the results of ureteropelvic junction surgery by diuresis renography. **a** Pre-pyeloplasty delayed IVP in a child who underwent prior abdominal exploration for pain demonstrates pyelocalyectasis without ureteral visualisation (gall bladder is opacified). Diuresis renography indicates obstruction to the right kidney; no obstruction on left.

Lasix at 15 min.   Lasix at 15 min.

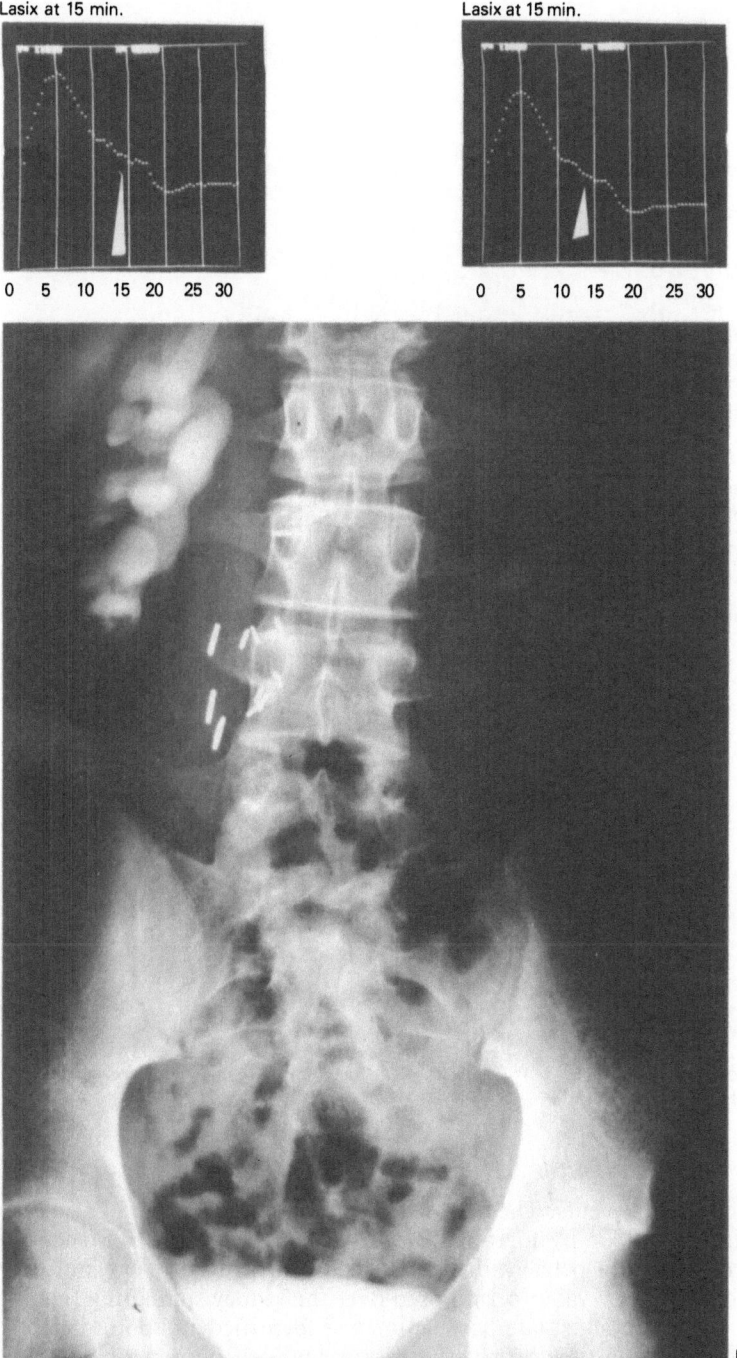

0   5   10 15 20 25 30   0   5   10 15   20   25 30

                                                                        b

Fig. 10.3b.   Thirteen days postoperatively the diuresis renogram became non-obstructed while the IVP was essentially unchanged.

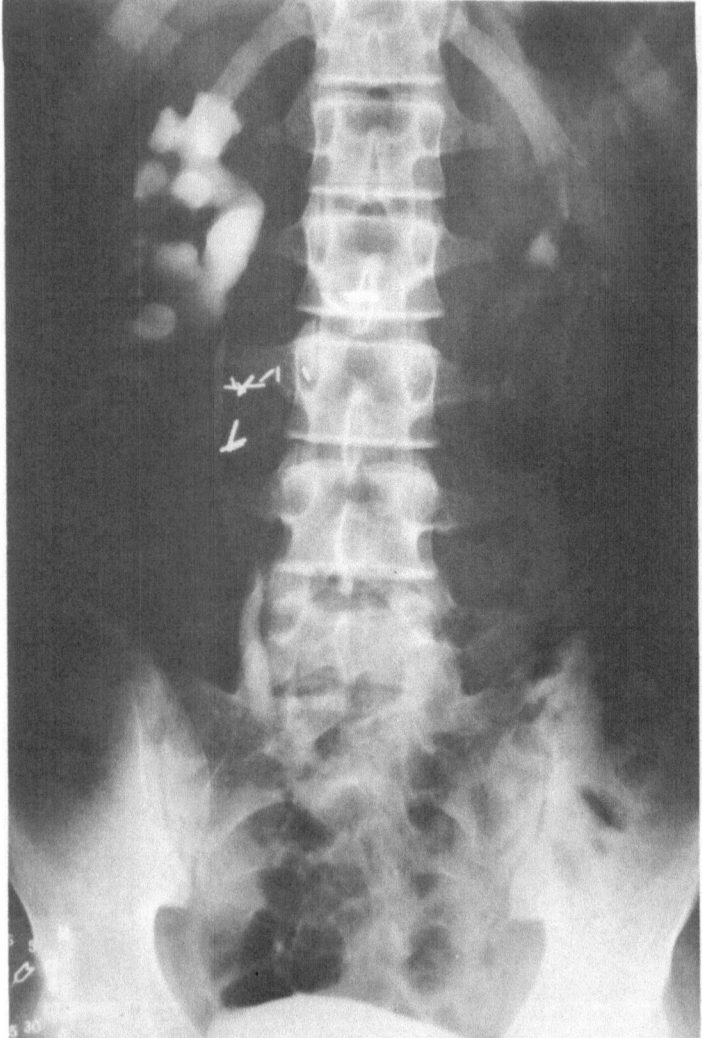

c

Fig. 10.3c. Late postoperative follow-up IVP (8 months) confirms improvement with appearance of contrast in ureter and diminished calyectasis.

years) were obtained in 25 patients. The non-obstructed pattern occurred in 22 cases and confirmed clinical and/or pyelographic improvement. Apparent obstruction was noted in one child with a pelvic kidney, but his result proved to be spurious because the distended bladder was superimposed over the kidney simulating failure of tracer washout. In two patients, late obstruction was identified and both patients required reoperation at which time obstructing fibrosis was encountered below the anastomotic site.

The operations performed are listed in Table 10.5. Primary nephrectomy was used in only two children whose thinned hydronephrotic kidneys displayed cystic changes. Seven adults with a mean age of 44 years also had primary nephrectomy because of irreparable renal damage. A temporary nephrostomy was used in only two cases with pyohydronephrosis.

Table 10.5. Operations

	No. of patients
Temporary nephrostomy	2
Lysis of adhesions	1
Disjoined pyeloureteroplasty	47
Pyeloureteroplasty — other types	11
Nephrectomy — primary	9
Re-operation	
Pyeloplasty	2
Drainage of urinoma	2
Nephrectomy	1

The most commonly performed operation was the Anderson-Hynes dismembered pyeloplasty. In children a stenting catheter and nephrostomy tube were used in almost all cases (Johnston et al. 1977). In adults, drainage alone without tubes or stents was preferred unless infection or scarring was observed.

Twenty patients diagnosed as having no significant obstruction were managed conservatively; 19 were adults of whom 12 were totally asymptomatic. Seven had varying degrees of intermittent flank pain judged preferable (by the patient) to the pain and risks of corrective surgery. None of these patients has since demonstrated progression of hydronephrosis nor required subsequent operation (Fig. 10.4).

The anatomical findings at the time of operation are recorded in Table 10.6. In each of the patients with massive reflux, the ureter was not narrowed but appeared either normal or dilated at the pelviureteric junction. In each case, sharp angulation caused the ureter to become progressively compressed against the renal pelvis as the latter increased in volume and became overdistended.

Table 10.6. Ureteropelvic junction pathology

	No. of kidneys
Angulation of ureter	7
Narrow segment	26
Vessel or band	12
Scar	4
Polyp	1
Multiple abnormalities	17

There was no operative mortality in this series. Delayed passage of urine across the anastomosis required retrograde ureteral catheterisation in three cases. A wound infection occurred once, and re-exploration to drain a urinoma was needed in two cases. All six complications occurred in patients in whom drainage alone was used. Reoperation with pyeloureteroplasty was required in two children after 1.5 and 2.5 years for radiographic deterioration and obstruction demonstrated by diuresis renography. Pathological findings in both cases were scar formation below the anastomosis which itself was intact; stenting with nephrostomy had been used in one

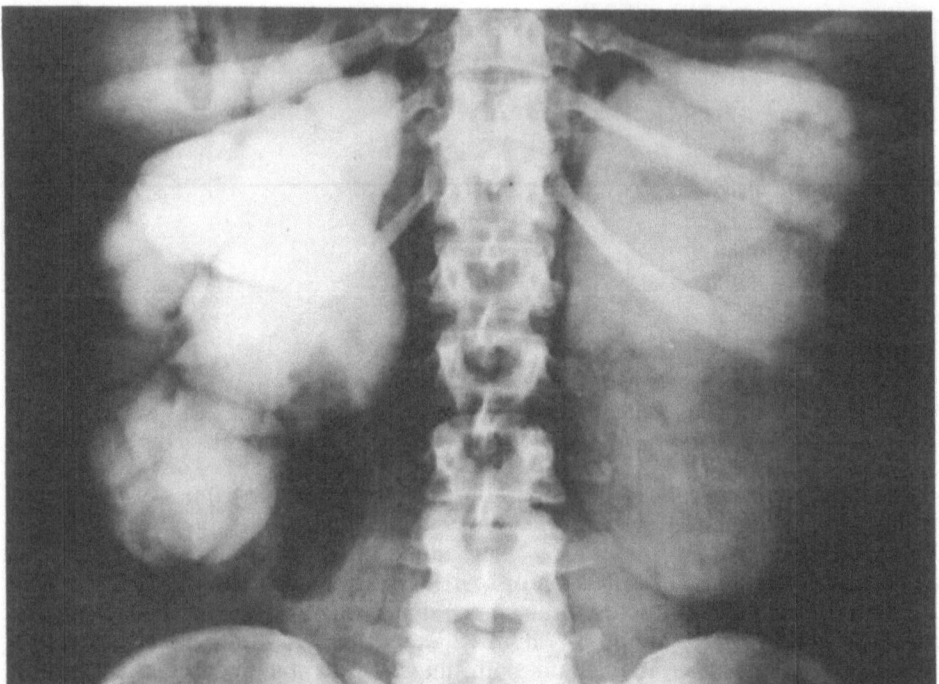

Fig. 10.4. Massive bilateral hydronephrosis remains unchanged in an asymptomatic 43-year-old woman with normal renal function (creatinine 0.7 mg%, BUN 9 mg%) who has been followed for 8 years without surgical intervention. Diuresis renography demonstrated a dilated but non-obstructed pattern on the right side and diminished function on the left.

case, drainage alone in the other. In one other case, a child in whom a temporary nephrostomy was placed for pyohydronephrosis, re-exploration revealed a contracted, scarred kidney with xanthogranulomatous pyelonephritis; nephrectomy was performed.

Except for one patient who was followed for only 8 months, all operated patients had a follow-up ranging 1–4 years. Some patients not operated upon have been followed for longer periods through the availability of prior radiographic studies. Patients operated for pain were all clinically improved. Radiographic improvement was defined as a reduction in the degree of calyceal dilation on IVP and occurred in 41 kidneys (69%). The calyces were unchanged in 16 kidneys and worse in two. Diuresis renography confirmed that there was no obstruction in 35 patients after operation and pressure flow measurements demonstrated operative success in four cases.

Discussion

The topic of idiopathic hydronephrosis has been comprehensively discussed in the standard urologic textbooks and in the recent literature (Drake et al. 1978; Hendren et al. 1980; Johnston et al. 1977; Snyder et al. 1980; Williams and Kenawi 1976;

Zincke et al. 1974). Little attention has been paid, however, to the indications for surgery, presumably due to the assumption that hydronephrosis was progressive, and because of difficulties in accurately defining and assessing partial obstruction. As a result it has been genuinely difficult to determine which patients, if any, with hydronephrosis do or do not require surgery.

In examining the indications for surgery at the present time, it is apparent that any pelviureteric junction abnormality requires surgical repair when serial IVP examination or other studies demonstrate progressive hydronephrosis or renal damage. Surgical intervention is likewise necessary whenever the newer diagnostic testing modalities (perfusion pressure flow or diuresis renography) establish the presence of a true obstruction. In the absence of definable obstruction or progressive obstructive damage, however, many patients will still require operative therapy because of symptoms or associated clinical features.

Painful hydronephrosis is one of the commonest patterns of presentation for this disease and an equally common indication for surgery. In its most severe form, associated with nausea, vomiting and a tense, tender abdominal mass, the need for surgical relief is definite. At the other end of the spectrum are patients with chronic lumbago and minimal calyceal distortion in whom the pathophysiologic connection between the two is dubious (as is the potential for improvement with surgery). Between these extremes are numerous patients with intermittent episodes of flank pain which often mimics gastrointestinal disease. Occasionally the kidney will appear normal and undilated between attacks and the actual diagnosis of hydronephrosis remains in question (Genereux and Monks 1972; Davies et al. 1978) (Fig. 10.5). In this setting a number of provocative diagnostic manoeuvres such as diuresis renography have been suggested and are often needed to establish the diagnosis (Kendall 1968). More commonly, variable degrees of hydronephrosis are observed on the IVP in the absence of pain, and at times during an episode of pain the dilatation worsens (Whitfield et al. 1979) (Fig. 10.6). After assessing obstruction in patients with painful hydronephrosis, ten adults in our series were identified in whom there was no evidence of obstruction in the absence of pain, and during attacks of pain which were infrequent, the discomfort was tolerable. We interpret these findings as indicating that except during episodes of pain, the kidney is not physiologically overdistended and is not in jeopardy from progressive hydronephrosis or renal damage: a state of equilibrium exists. All patients were offered non-operative management, trading occasional pain for the risks of surgery; eight patients chose this approach and none has subsequently required surgery nor demonstrated deterioration of renal function or pyelographic appearance.

Totally asymptomatic hydronephrosis is a disturbing entity, because it is evidence that on some previous occasions renal damage occurred silently. Undoubtedly, symptoms were present in many such patients but either occurred early in life or mimicked disturbances in other organ systems. Fourteen asymptomatic cases were identified in our series and all but one were adults with a mean age of 61 years. An IVU was repeated in the one child 6 months after diagnosis and progression of pelvicalyceal dilatation had silently occurred during the interval; pyeloplasty was therefore performed. Except for one adult who had a nephrectomy for a nonfunctioning kidney, the remaining 12 have been followed without operation. None has had evidence of obstruction and none has demonstrated progression of disease (Fig. 10.4).

In most of the children in this series a true obstruction was identified as the aetiology for hydronephrosis, which untreated was capable of progressing without symptoms. Silent progression of hydronephrosis in childhood has been recognised

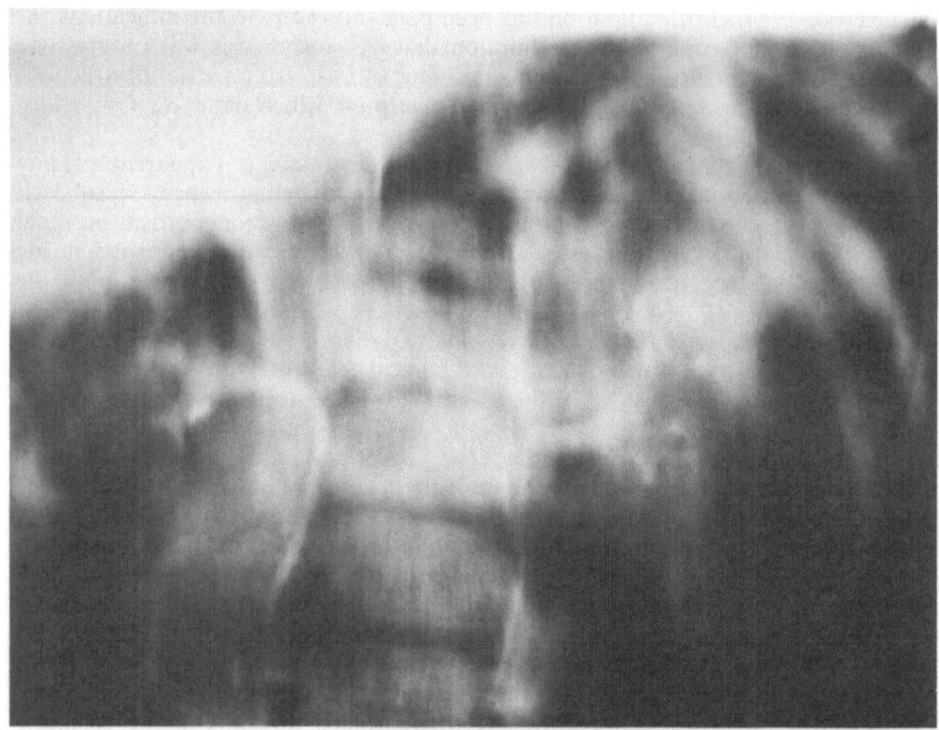

a

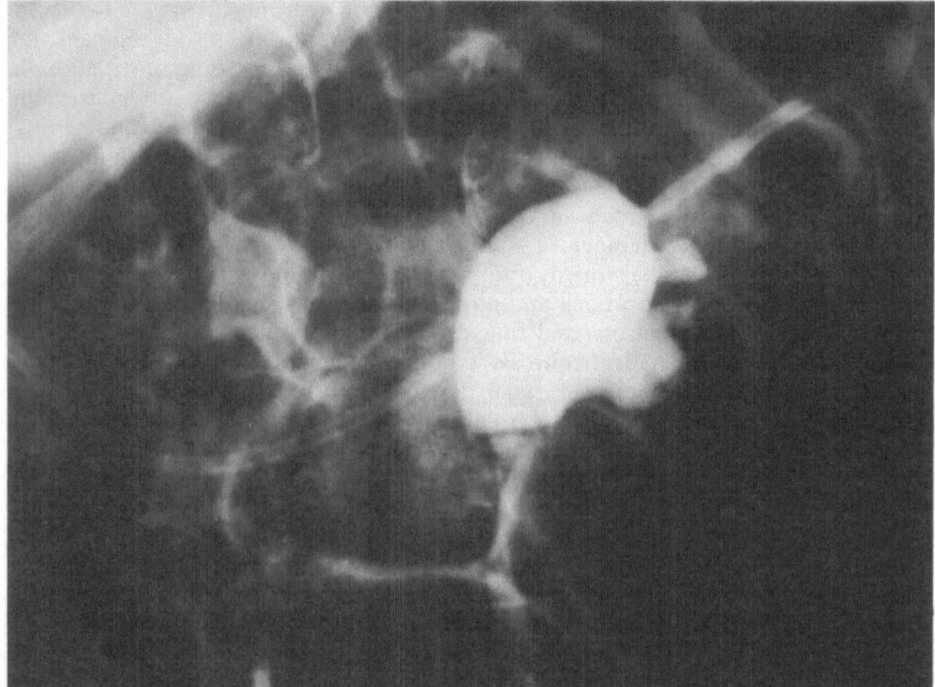

b

Fig. 10.5. Intermittent hydronephrosis: **a** IVP at 5 min demonstrates normal kidneys bilaterally. **b** IVP at 15 min reveals development of left hydronephrosis.

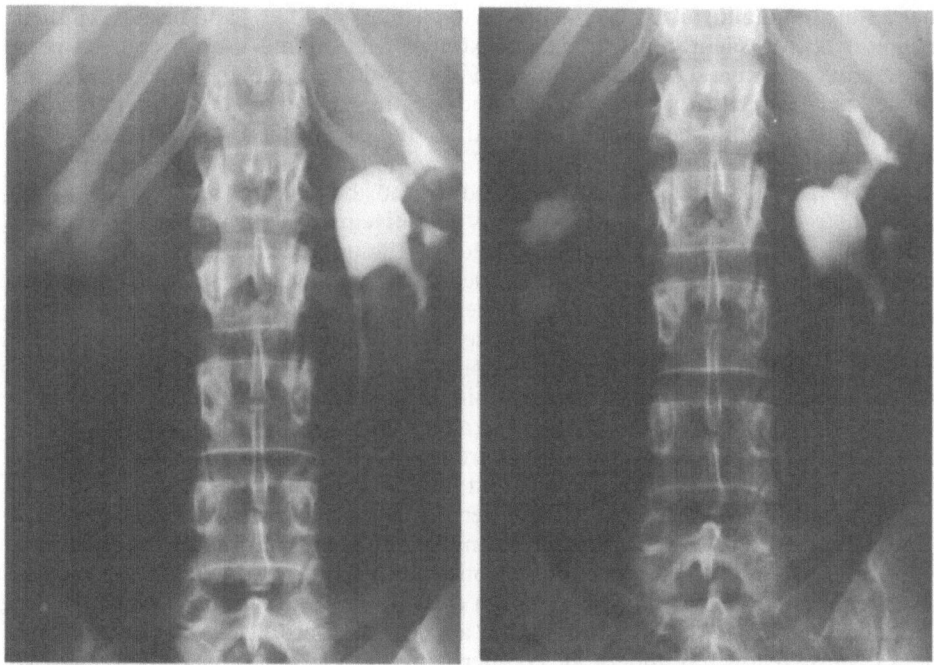

a   b

Fig. 10.6. Intermittent hydronephrosis: **a** IVP during an attack of pain shows right-sided hydronephrosis with poor visualisation. **b** IVP in the absence of pain reveals less dilatation.

and reported previously (McAllister et al. 1980). This contrasts sharply with the apparent lack of progression of hydronephrosis demonstrated in over 50% of the adults described above. Experimental evidence provides an explanation as to why hydronephrosis is less likely to progress in the adult kidney than in the paediatric kidney. In canine experiments, the measured physiologic capacity of the renal pelvis above which overdistension and high pressures occur was shown to increase in proportion to the size of the renal pelvis. In addition, once the pelvis was overdistended the rate at which pressures rose during volume expansion decreased (in an inverse exponential relationship) as the size of the renal pelvis became larger. As a result of these phenomena, the larger capacity pelvis requires more volume to become overdistended and once overdistended is subjected to a slower rate of overstretching and pressure increase than is the smaller pelvis. Consequently, an equilibrium state is more likely to occur in the large renal pelvis whenever physiologic fluctuations in diuresis provide insufficient volume expansion to overdistend the pelvis above capacity; therefore progression of hydronephrosis will not occur. The converse applies to the small capacity pelvis which may be subjected to rapidly increasing high pressures with only minimal increases in volume. The paediatric sized kidney, therefore, appears much more vulnerable to progression or hydronephrosis and parenchymal damage whenever it is subjected to volume expansion comparable to the adult kidney.

These preliminary observations suggest that a non-operative approach is feasible and safe in selected patients with hydronephrosis when selection is based on an accurate assessment of obstruction and is guided by an understanding of the pathophysiology of obstructive hydronephrosis. However, because it is less likely that a state of equilibrium is ever achieved in paediatric kidneys and because of their greater risk for silent renal damage, extreme caution must be exercised when considering non-operative management of idiopathic hydronephrosis in childhood.

The specifics of surgical technique and treatment of patients with idiopathic hydronephrosis have been well reviewed in the recent literature (Drake 1978; Hendren 1980; Johnston 1969; Johnston et al. 1972; Williams and Kenawi 1976; Snyder et al. 1980; Zincke et al. 1974) and will not be detailed herein.

One interesting problem which concerns operative management relates to kidneys which appear to be unsalvageable. In children, the unpredictable recoverability of the hydronephrotic kidney is well recognised and must govern any action (Zincke et al. 1974). Irreparable renal damage is often in the eyes of the beholder. IVP non-visualisation does not necessarily indicate poor future function especially in the newborn period when renal function is normally depressed. Likewise, at operation the kidney parenchyma may appear thin, but this can simply represent taut stretching of what will ultimately become adequate parenchyma over a tense fluid-filled sac; decompression may be rewarded by return of significant function. Finally, in reviewing our own patients and those in the literature, it is obvious that very little long term harm comes from performing a pyeloplasty in even the most hopelessly thinned kidney. Our nephrectomy rate of 4% in children is comparable to other recent series and supports this reconstructive philosophy; nephrectomy was never required after pyeloplasty (Hendren et al. 1980; Williams and Kenawi 1976). The same considerations probably do not apply to the chronically obstructed adult kidney whose fellow has undergone compensatory hypertrophy. Salvage of a poorly or non-functioning kidney in this setting is much less likely to be rewarded by improved function and often the patient can best be served by nephrectomy. The nephrectomy rate in our adult population was 20%.

Assessment of the result of surgery for pelviureteric junction obstruction is usually easy when the patient has symptoms such as flank pain, which are relieved postoperatively. It is difficult, however, to pathogenetically connect symptoms such as lower urinary tract infection and enuresis to hydronephrosis, and relief of these after operation should not be expected. Improvement in renal function is more difficult to confirm especially in the presence of a normally functioning or hypertrophied contralateral kidney; radionuclide techniques however may be helpful. In the past, postoperative evaluation was considered incomplete without an IVP to document anticipated improvement in hydronephrosis. Unfortunately, pyelographic improvement does not always occur and its significance depends on which portion of the kidney is scrutinised. If the overall size of the renal pelvis is measured, postoperative reduction may occur in almost all cases, especially if reduction pyeloplasty was performed concomitantly (Weber and Glenn 1970). When calyceal changes are specifically assessed, however, no improvement may be noted in a large number of patients (Johnston et al. 1977; Williams and Kenawi 1976).

Radiographic evaluation is further complicated by the fact that if the IVU is performed too soon after operation, it may demonstrate disturbing degrees of dilatation even after successful surgery. Maximal pyelographic improvement generally occurs between 6 to 12 months after operation (Johnston et al. 1977; Snyder et al. 1980). This unfortunately puts the clinician in the uncertain position of either accepting various degrees of hydronephrosis as a normal postoperative occurrence or abandoning early postoperative radiographic testing altogether. If a nephrostomy tube has been placed, it may be helpful in confirming anastomotic patency or be useful with perfusion studies in the early postoperative period (Snyder et al. 1980), but this is potentially stressful to the fresh anastomotic site.

Because of its ability to assess hydronephrosis and to distinguish between obstruction and non-obstructive dilatation, diuresis renography would seem to be a logical alternative to the IVU in examining the functional patency of the recently operated pelviureteric junction. A lower radiation dose is an added attraction. Experience in the present series confirms this usefulness. In 15 patients studied within 2 weeks of operation, no obstruction was noted in 13, while in two kidneys severe impairment in function precluded scan interpretation (Fig. 10.3). Diuresis renography was equally accurate in the late follow-up of surgical results, demonstrating no obstruction in 22 of 25 successfully treated patients. Two patients who required reoperation for late-occurring obstruction were initially identified by this technique. In one other case the result was falsely positive for obstruction because of accummulation of tracer in the distended bladder overlying an ectopic (pelvic) kidney. On the basis of these findings, the diuresis renogram appears currently to be the non-invasive diagnostic procedure of choice for the preoperative evaluation and the early and late follow-up of patients undergoing pyeloplasty.

The preceding discussion indicates that in providing the clinician with previously unavailable methods for accurately and reliably assessing urinary tract dilatation, these new diagnostic methods have demonstrated a major advance in the overall management of patients with idiopathic hydronephrosis. By recognising the pitfalls of each study and by integrating the results carefully, it will usually (but not always) be possible to establish a correct diagnosis and to arrive rationally at a therapeutic plan. Because these methods do not specifically measure the factors actually responsible for progression of hydronephrosis and renal damage, their results will at times be discordant. Until better tests are developed, however, we will have to settle for these empiric methods and to accept an occasional measure of inaccuracy.

References

Bratt CG, Aurell M, Nilsson S (1977) Renal function in patients with hydronephrosis. Br J Urol 49: 249

Davies P, Wood KA, Evans CM, Gray WM, Kulatilake AE (1978) The value of provocative and acute urography in patients with intermittent loin pain. Br J Urol 50: 227

Djurhuus JC, Dorph S, Christiansen C, Ladefoged O, Nerstrom B (1976) Predictive value of renography and I.V. urography for the outcome of reconstructive surgery in patients with hydronephrosis. Acta Chir Scand 472: 37

Drake DP, Stevens PS, Eckstein HB (1978) Hydronephrosis secondary to ureteropelvic obstruction in children: A review of 14 years of experience. J Urol 119: 649

Genereux GP, Monks JG (1972) Intermittent ureteropelvic junction obstruction: Pathophysiologic-radiologic features. J Can Assoc Radiol 23: 75

Hendren WH, Radhakrishman J, Middleton AW Jr (1980) Pediatric pyeloplasty. J Pediatr Surg 15: 113

Johnston JH (1969) The pathogenesis of hydronephrosis in children. Br J Urol 41: 724

Johnston JH, Kathel BL (1972) The results of surgery for hydronephrosis as determined by renography with analogue computer simulation. Br J Urol 44: 320

Johnston JH, Evans JP, Glassberg KI, Shapiro SR (1977) Pelvic hydronephrosis in children: A review of 219 personal cases. J Urol 117: 97

Kendall AR, Karafin L (1968) Intermittent hydronephrosis: Hydration pyelography. J Urol 98: 653

Krueger RP, Ash JM, Silver MM, Kass EJ, Gilmour RJ, Alton DJ, Gilday DL, Churchill BM (1980) Primary hydronephrosis. Urol Clin North Am 7: 231

McAllister WH, Manley CB, Siegel MJ (1980) Asymptomatic progression of partial ureteropelvic obstruction in children. J Urol 123: 267

Nilsson S, Aurell M, Bratt CG (1979) Maximum urinary concentration ability in patients with idiopathic hydronephrosis. Br J Urol 51: 432

Roberts JBM, Slade N (1964) The natural history of primary pelvic hydronephrosis. Br J Surg 51: 759

Snyder HM, Lebowitz RL, Colodmy AH, Bauer SB, Retik AB (1980) Ureteropelvic junction obstruction in children. Urol Clin North Am 7: 273

Wax SH, McDonald DF (1966) The renogram vs the pyelogram: Evaluation of the significance of upper urinary tract obstruction. J Urol 96: 816

Weber CH, Glenn JF (1970) Hydronephrosis due to ureteropelvic junction obstruction: The efficacy of pyeloplastic surgery. Am Surg 36: 69

Whitaker RH (1977) Hydronephrosis. Ann R Coll Surg Engl 59: 388

Whitaker RH (1978) Clinical assessment of pelvic and ureteral function. Urology 12: 146

Whitfield HN, Britton KE, Hendry WF, Wickham JEA (1979) Furosemide intravenous urography in the diagnosis of pelviureteric junction obstruction. Br J Urol 51: 445

Williams DI, Kenawi MM (1976) The prognosis of pelviureteric obstruction in childhood. Eur Urol 2: 57

Zincke H, Kelalis PP, Culp OS (1974) Ureteropelvic obstruction in children. Surg Gynecol Obstet 139: 873

Subject Index